How To Control Diabetes And Improve Your Quality Of Life

321 Great Tips To Successfully Manage Your Diabetes

ADAM COLTON

Published by BizMove
www.bizmove.com

ISBN: 1978399804
ISBN- 978-1978399808

Table of Contents

ADAM COLTON

1. Diabetes Fact Sheet

What is Diabetes?

Diabetes is a disease that occurs when your blood glucose, also called blood sugar, is too high. Blood glucose is your main source of energy and comes from the food you eat. Insulin, a hormone made by the pancreas, helps glucose from food get into your cells to be used for energy. Sometimes your body doesn't make enough—or any—insulin or doesn't use insulin well. Glucose then stays in your blood and doesn't reach your cells.

Over time, having too much glucose in your blood can cause health problems. Although diabetes has no cure, you can take steps to manage your diabetes and stay healthy.

Sometimes people call diabetes "a touch of sugar" or "borderline diabetes." These terms suggest that someone doesn't really have diabetes or has a less serious case, but every case of diabetes is serious.

What are the different types of diabetes?

The most common types of diabetes are type 1, type 2, and gestational diabetes.

Type 1 diabetes

If you have type 1 diabetes, your body does not make insulin. Your immune system attacks and destroys the cells in your pancreas that make insulin. Type 1 diabetes is usually diagnosed in children and young adults, although it can appear at any age. People with type 1 diabetes need to take insulin every day to stay alive.

Type 2 diabetes

If you have type 2 diabetes, your body does not make or use insulin well. You can develop type 2 diabetes at any age, even during childhood. However, this type of diabetes occurs most often in middle-aged and older people. Type 2 is the most common type of diabetes.

Gestational diabetes

Gestational diabetes develops in some women when they are pregnant. Most of the time, this type of diabetes goes away after the baby is born. However, if you've had gestational diabetes, you have a greater chance of developing type 2 diabetes later in life. Sometimes diabetes diagnosed during pregnancy is actually type 2 diabetes.

Other types of diabetes

Less common types include monogenic diabetes, which is an inherited form of diabetes, and cystic fibrosis-related diabetes .

How common is diabetes?

About 30 million people in the United States, or 9.4 percent of the population, had diabetes. More than 1 in 4 of them didn't know they had the disease. Diabetes affects 1 in 4 people over the age of 65. About 90-95 percent of cases in adults are type 2 diabetes.[1]

Who is more likely to develop type 2 diabetes?

You are more likely to develop type 2 diabetes if you are age 45 or older, have a family history of diabetes, or are overweight. Physical inactivity, race, and certain health problems such as high blood pressure also affect your chance of developing type 2 diabetes. You are also more likely to develop type 2 diabetes if you have prediabetes or had gestational diabetes when you were pregnant. Learn more about risk factors for type 2 diabetes.

What health problems can people with diabetes develop?

Over time, high blood glucose leads to problems such as

- heart disease
- stroke
- kidney disease
- eye problems
- dental disease
- nerve damage
- foot problems

Symptoms & Causes of Diabetes

What are the symptoms of diabetes?

Symptoms of diabetes include

- increased thirst and urination
- increased hunger
- fatigue
- blurred vision
- numbness or tingling in the feet or hands
- sores that do not heal
- unexplained weight loss

Symptoms of type 1 diabetes can start quickly, in a matter of weeks. Symptoms of type 2 diabetes often develop slowly—over the course of several years—and can be so mild that you might not even notice them. Many people with type 2 diabetes have no symptoms. Some people do not find out they have the disease until they have diabetes-related health problems, such as blurred vision or heart trouble.

What causes type 1 diabetes?

Type 1 diabetes occurs when your immune system, the body's system for fighting infection, attacks and destroys the insulin-producing beta cells of the pancreas. Scientists think type 1 diabetes is caused by genes and environmental factors, such as viruses, that might trigger the disease.

What causes type 2 diabetes?

Type 2 diabetes—the most common form of diabetes—is caused by several factors, including lifestyle factors and genes.

Overweight, obesity, and physical inactivity

You are more likely to develop type 2 diabetes if you are not physically active and are overweight or obese. Extra weight sometimes causes insulin resistance and is common in people with type 2 diabetes. The location of body fat also makes a difference. Extra belly fat is linked to insulin resistance, type 2 diabetes, and heart and blood vessel disease. To see if your weight puts you at risk for type 2 diabetes, check out these Body Mass Index (BMI) charts.

Insulin resistance

Type 2 diabetes usually begins with insulin resistance, a condition in which muscle, liver, and fat cells do not use insulin well. As a result, your body needs more insulin to help glucoseenter cells. At first, the pancreas makes more insulin to keep up with the added demand. Over time, the pancreas can't make enough insulin, and blood glucose levels rise.

Genes and family history

As in type 1 diabetes, certain genes may make you more likely to develop type 2 diabetes. The disease tends to run in families and occurs more often in these racial/ethnic groups:

- African Americans
- Alaska Natives
- American Indians
- Asian Americans
- Hispanics/Latinos

- Native Hawaiians
- Pacific Islanders

Genes also can increase the risk of type 2 diabetes by increasing a person's tendency to become overweight or obese.

What causes gestational diabetes?

Scientists believe gestational diabetes, a type of diabetes that develops during pregnancy, is caused by the hormonal changes of pregnancy along with genetic and lifestyle factors.

Insulin resistance

Hormones produced by the placenta contribute to insulin resistance, which occurs in all women during late pregnancy. Most pregnant women can produce enough insulin to overcome insulin resistance, but some cannot. Gestational diabetes occurs when the pancreas can't make enough insulin.

As with type 2 diabetes, extra weight is linked to gestational diabetes. Women who are overweight or obese may already have insulin resistance when they become pregnant. Gaining too much weight during pregnancy may also be a factor.

Genes and family history

Having a family history of diabetes makes it more likely that a woman will develop gestational diabetes, which suggests that genes play a role. Genes may also explain why the disorder occurs more often in African Americans, American Indians, Asians, and Hispanics/Latinas.

What else can cause diabetes?

Genetic mutations , other diseases, damage to the pancreas, and certain medicines may also cause diabetes.

Genetic mutations

- Monogenic diabetes is caused by mutations, or changes, in a single gene. These changes are usually passed through families, but sometimes the gene mutation happens on its own. Most of these gene mutations cause diabetes by making the pancreas less able to make insulin. The most common types of monogenic diabetes are neonatal diabetes and maturity-onset diabetes of the young (MODY). Neonatal diabetes occurs in the first 6 months of life. Doctors usually diagnose MODY during adolescence or early adulthood, but sometimes the disease is not diagnosed until later in life.

- Cystic fibrosis produces thick mucus that causes scarring in the pancreas. This scarring can prevent the pancreas from making enough insulin.
- Hemochromatosis causes the body to store too much iron. If the disease is not treated, iron can build up in and damage the pancreas and other organs.

Hormonal diseases

Some hormonal diseases cause the body to produce too much of certain hormones, which sometimes cause insulin resistance and diabetes.

- Cushing's syndrome occurs when the body produces too much cortisol—often called the "stress hormone."
- Acromegaly occurs when the body produces too much growth hormone.
- Hyperthyroidism occurs when the thyroid gland produces too much thyroid hormone.

Damage to or removal of the pancreas

Pancreatitis, pancreatic cancer, and trauma can all harm the beta cells or make them less able to produce insulin, resulting in diabetes. If the damaged pancreas is removed, diabetes will occur due to the loss of the beta cells.

Medicines

Sometimes certain medicines can harm beta cells or disrupt the way insulin works. These include

- niacin, a type of vitamin B3
- certain types of diuretics, also called water pills
- anti-seizure drugs
- psychiatric drugs
- drugs to treat human immunodeficiency virus (HIV)
- pentamidine, a drug used to treat a type of pneumonia
- glucocorticoids—medicines used to treat inflammatory illnesses such as rheumatoid arthritis , asthma , lupus , and ulcerative colitis
- anti-rejection medicines, used to help stop the body from rejecting a transplanted organ

Statins, which are medicines to reduce LDL ("bad") cholesterol levels, can slightly increase the chance that you'll develop diabetes. However, statins help protect you from heart disease and stroke. For this reason, the strong benefits of taking statins outweigh the small chance that you could develop diabetes.

If you take any of these medicines and are concerned about their side effects, talk with your doctor.

Managing Diabetes

You can manage your diabetes and live a long and healthy life by taking care of yourself each day.

Diabetes can affect almost every part of your body. Therefore, you will need to manage your blood glucose levels, also called blood sugar. Managing your blood glucose, as well as your blood pressure and cholesterol, can help prevent the health problems that can occur when you have diabetes.

How can I manage my diabetes?

With the help of your health care team, you can create a diabetes self-care plan to manage your diabetes. Your self-care plan may include these steps:

Ways to manage your diabetes
- Manage your diabetes ABCs.
- Follow your diabetes meal plan.
- Make physical activity part of your routine.
- Take your medicine.
- Check your blood glucose levels.

- Work with your health care team.
- Cope with your diabetes in healthy ways.

Manage your diabetes ABCs

Knowing your diabetes ABCs will help you manage your blood glucose, blood pressure, and cholesterol. Stopping smoking if you smoke will also help you manage your diabetes. Working toward your ABC goals can help lower your chances of having a heart attack, stroke, or other diabetes problems.

A for the A1C test

The A1C test shows your average blood glucose level over the past 3 months. The A1C goal for many people with diabetes is below 7 percent. Ask your health care team what your goal should be.

B for Blood pressure

The blood pressure goal for most people with diabetes is below 140/90 mm Hg. Ask what your goal should be.

C for Cholesterol

You have two kinds of cholesterol in your blood: LDL and HDL. LDL or "bad" cholesterol can build up and clog your blood vessels. Too much bad cholesterol can cause a heart attack or stroke. HDL or "good" cholesterol helps remove the "bad" cholesterol from your blood vessels.

Ask your health care team what your cholesterol numbers should be. If you are over 40 years of age, you may need to take a statin drug for heart health.

S for Stop smoking

Not smoking is especially important for people with diabetes because both smoking and diabetes narrow blood vessels. Blood vessel narrowing makes your heart work harder. E-cigarettes aren't a safe option either.

If you quit smoking

- you will lower your risk for heart attack, stroke, nerve disease, kidney disease, diabetic eye disease, and amputation
- your cholesterol and blood pressure levels may improve
- your blood circulation will improve
- you may have an easier time being physically active

If you smoke or use other tobacco products, stop. Ask for help so you don't have to do it alone. You can start by calling the national quitline at 1-800-

QUITNOW or 1-800-784-8669. For tips on quitting, go to SmokeFree.gov .

Keeping your A1C, blood pressure, and cholesterol levels close to your goals and stopping smoking may help prevent the long-term harmful effects of diabetes. These health problems include heart disease, stroke, kidney disease, nerve damage, and eye disease. You can keep track of your ABCs with a diabetes care record (PDF, 568 KB). Take it with you on your health care visits. Talk about your goals and how you are doing, and whether you need to make any changes in your diabetes care plan.

Follow your diabetes meal plan

Make a diabetes meal plan with help from your health care team. Following a meal plan will help you manage your blood glucose, blood pressure, and cholesterol.

Choose fruits and vegetables, beans, whole grains, chicken or turkey without the skin, fish, lean meats, and nonfat or low-fat milk and cheese. Drink water instead of sugar-sweetened beverages. Choose foods that are lower in calories, saturated fat, trans fat, sugar, and salt. Learn more about eating, diet, and nutrition with diabetes.

Make physical activity part of your daily routine

Set a goal to be more physically active. Try to work up to 30 minutes or more of physical activity on most days of the week.

Brisk walking and swimming are good ways to move more. If you are not active now, ask your health care team about the types and amounts of physical activity that are right for you. Learn more about being physically active with diabetes.

Following your meal plan and being more active can help you stay at or get to a healthy weight. If you are overweight or obese, work with your health care team to create a weight-loss plan that is right for you.

Take your medicine

Take your medicines for diabetes and any other health problems, even when you feel good or have reached your blood glucose, blood pressure, and cholesterol goals. These medicines help you manage your ABCs. Ask your doctor if you need to take aspirin to prevent a heart attack or stroke. Tell your health care professional if you cannot afford your medicines or if you have any side effects from your medicines. Learn more about insulin and other diabetes medicines.

Check your blood glucose levels

For many people with diabetes, checking their blood glucose level each day is an important way to manage their diabetes. Monitoring your blood glucose level is most important if you take insulin. The results of blood glucose monitoring can help you make decisions about food, physical activity, and medicines.

The most common way to check your blood glucose level at home is with a blood glucose meter. You get a drop of blood by pricking the side of your fingertip with a lancet. Then you apply the blood to a test strip. The meter will show you how much glucose is in your blood at the moment.

Ask your health care team how often you should check your blood glucose levels. Make sure to keep a record of your blood glucose self-checks. You can print copies of this glucose self-check chart (PDF, 2 MB). Take these records with you when you visit your health care team.

What is continuous glucose monitoring?

Continuous glucose monitoring (CGM) is another way to check your glucose levels. Most CGM systems use a tiny sensor that you insert under your skin. The sensor measures glucose levels in the fluids between your body's cells every few minutes and can show changes in your glucose level throughout the day and night. If the CGM system shows that your glucose is too high or too low, you should check your glucose with a blood glucose meter before making any changes to your eating plan, physical activity, or medicines. A CGM system is especially useful for people who use insulin and have problems with low blood glucose.

What are the recommended targets for blood glucose levels?

Many people with diabetes aim to keep their blood glucose at these normal levels:

- Before a meal: 80 to 130 mg/dL
- About 2 hours after a meal starts: less than 180 mg/dL

Talk with your health care team about the best target range for you. Be sure to tell your health care professional if your glucose levels often go above or below your target range.

What happens if my blood glucose level becomes too low?

Sometimes blood glucose levels drop below where they should be, which is called hypoglycemia. For most people with diabetes, the blood glucose level is too low when it is below 70 mg/dL.

Hypoglycemia can be life threatening and needs to be treated right away.

What happens if my blood glucose level becomes too high?

Doctors call high blood glucose hyperglycemia.

Symptoms that your blood glucose levels may be too high include

- feeling thirsty
- feeling tired or weak
- headaches
- urinating often
- blurred vision

If you often have high blood glucose levels or symptoms of high blood glucose, talk with your health care team. You may need a change in your diabetes meal plan, physical activity plan, or medicines.

Know when to check for ketones

Your doctor may want you to check your urine for ketones if you have symptoms of diabetic ketoacidosis . When ketone levels get too high, you can develop this life-threatening condition. Symptoms include

- trouble breathing
- nausea or vomiting
- pain in your abdomen
- confusion
- feeling very tired or sleepy

Ketoacidosis most often is a problem for people with type 1 diabetes.

Work with your health care team

Most people with diabetes get health care from a primary care professional. Primary care professionals include internists, family physicians, and pediatricians. Sometimes physician assistants and nurses with extra training, called nurse practitioners, provide primary care. You also will need to see other care professionals from time to time. A team of health care professionals can help you improve your diabetes self-care. Remember, you are the most important member of your health care team.

Besides a primary care professional, your health care team may include

- an endocrinologist for more specialized diabetes care
- a registered dietitian, also called a nutritionist
- a nurse
- a certified diabetes educator
- a pharmacist
- a dentist
- an eye doctor
- a podiatrist, or foot doctor, for foot care
- a social worker, who can help you find financial aid for treatment and community resources
- a counselor or other mental health care professional

When you see members of your health care team, ask questions. Write a list of questions you have before your visit so you don't forget what you want to ask.

You should see your health care team at least twice a year, and more often if you are having problems or are having trouble reaching your blood glucose, blood pressure, or cholesterol goals. At each visit, be sure you have a blood pressure check, foot check, and weight check; and review your self-care plan. Talk with your health care team about your medicines and whether you need to adjust them. Routine health care will help you find and treat any health problems early, or may be able to help prevent them.

Talk with your doctor about what vaccines you should get to keep from getting sick, such as a flu shot and pneumonia shot. Preventing illness is an important part of taking care of your diabetes. Your blood glucose levels are more likely to go up when you're sick or have an infection.

Cope with your diabetes in healthy ways

Feeling stressed, sad, or angry is common when you live with diabetes. Stress can raise your blood glucose levels, but you can learn ways to lower your stress. Try deep breathing, gardening, taking a walk, doing yoga, meditating, doing a hobby, or listening to your favorite music. Consider taking part in a diabetes education program or support group that teaches you techniques for managing stress.

Depression is common among people with a chronic, or long-term, illness . Depression can get in the way of your efforts to manage your diabetes. Ask for help if you feel down. A mental health counselor, support group, clergy member, friend, or family member who will listen to your feelings may help you feel better.

Try to get 7 to 8 hours of sleep each night. Getting enough sleep can help improve your mood and energy level. You can take steps to improve your sleep habits . If you often feel sleepy during the day, you may have obstructive sleep apnea , a condition in which your breathing briefly stops many times during the night. Sleep apnea is common in people who have diabetes. Talk with your health care team if you think you have a sleep problem.

Diabetes Diet, Eating, & Physical Activity

Nutrition and physical activity are important parts of a healthy lifestyle when you have diabetes. Along with other benefits, following a healthy meal plan and being active can help you keep your blood glucose level, also called blood sugar, in your target range. To manage your blood glucose, you need to balance what you eat and drink with physical activity and diabetes medicine, if you take any. What you choose to eat, how much you eat, and when you eat are all important in keeping your blood glucose level in the range that your health care team recommends.

Becoming more active and making changes in what you eat and drink can seem challenging at first. You may find it easier to start with small changes and get help from your family, friends, and health care team.

Eating well and being physically active most days of the week can help you

- keep your blood glucose level, blood pressure, and cholesterol in your target ranges
- lose weight or stay at a healthy weight
- prevent or delay diabetes problems
- feel good and have more energy

What foods can I eat if I have diabetes?

You may worry that having diabetes means going without foods you enjoy. The good news is that you can still eat your favorite foods, but you might need to eat smaller portions or enjoy them less often. Your health care team will help create a diabetes meal plan for you that meets your needs and likes.

The key to eating with diabetes is to eat a variety of healthy foods from all food groups, in the amounts your meal plan outlines.

The food groups are

- **vegetables**
- nonstarchy: includes broccoli, carrots, greens, peppers, and tomatoes
- starchy: includes potatoes, corn, and green peas
- **fruits**—includes oranges, melon, berries, apples, bananas, and grapes

- **grains**—at least half of your grains for the day should be whole grains
- includes wheat, rice, oats, cornmeal, barley, and quinoa
- examples: bread, pasta, cereal, and tortillas
- **protein**
- lean meat
- chicken or turkey without the skin
- fish
- eggs
- nuts and peanuts
- dried beans and certain peas, such as chickpeas and split peas
- meat substitutes, such as tofu
- **dairy—nonfat or low fat**
- milk or lactose-free milk if you have lactose intolerance
- yogurt
- cheese

Eat foods with heart-healthy fats, which mainly come from these foods:

- oils that are liquid at room temperature, such as canola and olive oil
- nuts and seeds
- heart-healthy fish such as salmon, tuna, and mackerel

- avocado

Use oils when cooking food instead of butter, cream, shortening, lard, or stick margarine.

What foods and drinks should I limit if I have diabetes?

Foods and drinks to limit include

- fried foods and other foods high in saturated fat and trans fat
- foods high in salt, also called sodium
- sweets, such as baked goods, candy, and ice cream
- beverages with added sugars, such as juice, regular soda, and regular sports or energy drinks

Drink water instead of sweetened beverages. Consider using a sugar substitute in your coffee or tea.

If you drink alcohol, drink moderately—no more than one drink a day if you're a woman or two drinks a day if you're a man. If you use insulin or diabetes medicines that increase the amount of insulin your body makes, alcohol can make your blood glucose level drop too low. This is especially true if you haven't eaten in a while. It's best to eat some food when you drink alcohol.

When should I eat if I have diabetes?

Some people with diabetes need to eat at about the same time each day. Others can be more flexible with the timing of their meals. Depending on your diabetes medicines or type of insulin, you may need to eat the same amount of carbohydrates at the same time each day. If you take "mealtime" insulin, your eating schedule can be more flexible.

If you use certain diabetes medicines or insulin and you skip or delay a meal, your blood glucose level can drop too low. Ask your health care team when you should eat and whether you should eat before and after physical activity.

How much can I eat if I have diabetes?

Eating the right amount of food will also help you manage your blood glucose level and your weight. Your health care team can help you figure out how much food and how many calories you should eat each day.

Weight-loss planning

If you are overweight or obese, work with your health care team to create a weight-loss plan.

To lose weight, you need to eat fewer calories and replace less healthy foods with foods lower in calories, fat, and sugar.

If you have diabetes, are overweight or obese, and are planning to have a baby, you should try to lose any excess weight before you become pregnant.

Meal plan methods

Two common ways to help you plan how much to eat if you have diabetes are the plate method and carbohydrate counting, also called carb counting. Check with your health care team about the method that's best for you.

Plate method

The plate method helps you control your portion sizes. You don't need to count calories. The plate method shows the amount of each food group you should eat. This method works best for lunch and dinner.

Use a 9-inch plate. Put nonstarchy vegetables on half of the plate; a meat or other protein on one-fourth of the plate; and a grain or other starch on the last one-fourth. Starches include starchy vegetables such as corn and peas. You also may eat a small bowl of fruit or a piece of fruit, and drink a small glass of milk as included in your meal plan.

You can find many different combinations of food and more details about using the plate method from the American Diabetes Association's Create Your Plate .

Your daily eating plan also may include small snacks between meals.

Portion sizes

- You can use everyday objects or your hand to judge the size of a portion.
- 1 serving of meat or poultry is the palm of your hand or a deck of cards
- 1 3-ounce serving of fish is a checkbook
- 1 serving of cheese is six dice
- 1/2 cup of cooked rice or pasta is a rounded handful or a tennis ball
- 1 serving of a pancake or waffle is a DVD
- 2 tablespoons of peanut butter is a ping-pong ball

Carbohydrate counting

Carbohydrate counting involves keeping track of the amount of carbohydrates you eat and drink each day. Because carbohydrates turn into glucose in your body, they affect your blood glucose level more than other foods do. Carb counting can help you manage your blood glucose level. If you take insulin, counting carbohydrates can help you know how much insulin to take.

The right amount of carbohydrates varies by how you manage your diabetes, including how physically active you are and what medicines you take, if any. Your health care team can help you create a personal eating plan based on carbohydrate counting.

The amount of carbohydrates in foods is measured in grams. To count carbohydrate grams in what you eat, you'll need to

- learn which foods have carbohydrates
- read the Nutrition Facts food label, or learn to estimate the number of grams of carbohydrate in the foods you eat
- add the grams of carbohydrate from each food you eat to get your total for each meal and for the day

Most carbohydrates come from starches, fruits, milk, and sweets. Try to limit carbohydrates with added sugars or those with refined grains, such as white bread and white rice. Instead, eat carbohydrates from fruit, vegetables, whole grains, beans, and low-fat or nonfat milk.

In addition to using the plate method and carb counting, you may want to visit a registered dietitian (RD) for medical nutrition therapy.

What is medical nutrition therapy?

Medical nutrition therapy is a service provided by an RD to create personal eating plans based on your needs and likes. For people with diabetes, medical nutrition therapy has been shown to improve diabetes management. Medicare pays for medical nutrition therapy for people with diabetes. If you have insurance other than Medicare, ask if it covers medical nutrition therapy for diabetes.

Will supplements and vitamins help my diabetes?

No clear proof exists that taking dietary supplements such as vitamins, minerals, herbs, or spices can help manage diabetes.[1] You may need supplements if you cannot get enough vitamins and minerals from foods. Talk with your health care provider before you take any dietary supplement since some can cause side effects or affect how your medicines work.[2]

Why should I be physically active if I have diabetes?

Physical activity is an important part of managing your blood glucose level and staying healthy. Being active has many health benefits.

Physical activity

- lowers blood glucose levels
- lowers blood pressure
- improves blood flow
- burns extra calories so you can keep your weight down if needed
- improves your mood
- can prevent falls and improve memory in older adults
- may help you sleep better

If you are overweight, combining physical activity with a reduced-calorie eating plan can lead to even more benefits. In the Look AHEAD: Action for Health in Diabetes study, overweight adults with type 2 diabetes who ate less and moved more had greater long-term health benefits compared to those who didn't make these changes. These benefits included improved cholesterol levels, less sleep apnea, and being able to move around more easily.

Even small amounts of physical activity can help. Experts suggest that you aim for at least 30 minutes of moderate or vigorous physical activity 5 days of the week.[3] Moderate activity feels somewhat hard, and vigorous activity is intense and feels hard. If you want to lose weight or maintain weight loss, you may need to do 60 minutes or more of physical activity 5 days of the week.

Be patient. It may take a few weeks of physical activity before you see changes in your health.

How can I be physically active safely if I have diabetes?

Be sure to drink water before, during, and after exercise to stay well hydrated. The following are some other tips for safe physical activity when you have diabetes.

Plan ahead

Talk with your health care team before you start a new physical activity routine, especially if you have other health problems. Your health care team will tell you a target range for your blood glucose level and suggest how you can be active safely.

Your health care team also can help you decide the best time of day for you to do physical activity based on your daily schedule, meal plan, and diabetes medicines. If you take insulin, you need to balance the activity that you do with your insulin doses and meals so you don't get low blood glucose.

Prevent low blood glucose

Because physical activity lowers your blood glucose, you should protect yourself against low blood glucose levels, also called hypoglycemia. You are most likely to have hypoglycemia if you take insulin or certain other diabetes medicines, such as a sulfonylurea. Hypoglycemia also can occur after a long intense workout or if you have skipped a meal before being active. Hypoglycemia can happen during or up to 24 hours after physical activity.

Planning is key to preventing hypoglycemia. For instance, if you take insulin, your health care provider might suggest you take less insulin or eat a small snack with carbohydrates before, during, or after physical activity, especially intense activity.[4]

You may need to check your blood glucose level before, during, and right after you are physically active.

Stay safe when blood glucose is high

If you have type 1 diabetes, avoid vigorous physical activity when you have ketones in your blood or urine. Ketones are chemicals your body might make when your blood glucose level is too high, a condition called hyperglycemia, and your insulin level is too low. If you are physically active when you have ketones in your blood or urine, your blood glucose level may go even higher. Ask your health care team what level of ketones are dangerous for you and how to test for them. Ketones are uncommon in people with type 2 diabetes.

Take care of your feet

People with diabetes may have problems with their feet because of poor blood flow and nerve damage that can result from high blood glucose levels. To help prevent foot problems, you should wear comfortable, supportive shoes and take care of your feet before, during, and after physical activity.

What physical activities should I do if I have diabetes?

Most kinds of physical activity can help you take care of your diabetes. Certain activities may be unsafe for some people, such as those with low vision or nerve damage to their feet. Ask your health care team what physical activities are safe for you. Many people choose walking with friends or family members for their activity.

Doing different types of physical activity each week will give you the most health benefits. Mixing it up also helps reduce boredom and lower your chance of getting hurt. Try these options for physical activity.

Add extra activity to your daily routine

If you have been inactive or you are trying a new activity, start slowly, with 5 to 10 minutes a day. Then add a little more time each week. Increase daily activity by spending less time in front of a TV or other screen. Try these simple ways to add physical activities in your life each day:

- Walk around while you talk on the phone or during TV commercials.
- Do chores, such as work in the garden, rake leaves, clean the house, or wash the car.
- Park at the far end of the shopping center parking lot and walk to the store.
- Take the stairs instead of the elevator.
- Make your family outings active, such as a family bike ride or a walk in a park.

If you are sitting for a long time, such as working at a desk or watching TV, do some light activity for 3 minutes or more every half hour.[5] Light activities include

- leg lifts or extensions
- overhead arm stretches
- desk chair swivels
- torso twists
- side lunges
- walking in place

Do aerobic exercise

Aerobic exercise is activity that makes your heart beat faster and makes you breathe harder. You should aim for doing aerobic exercise for 30 minutes a day most days of the week. You do not have to do all the activity at one time. You can split up these minutes into a few times throughout the day.

To get the most out of your activity, exercise at a moderate to vigorous level. Try

- walking briskly or hiking
- climbing stairs
- swimming or a water-aerobics class
- dancing
- riding a bicycle or a stationary bicycle
- taking an exercise class
- playing basketball, tennis, or other sports

Talk with your health care team about how to warm up and cool down before and after you exercise.

Do strength training to build muscle

Strength training is a light or moderate physical activity that builds muscle and helps keep your bones healthy. Strength training is important for both men and women. When you have more muscle and less body fat, you'll burn more calories. Burning more calories can help you lose and keep off extra weight.

You can do strength training with hand weights, elastic bands, or weight machines. Try to do strength training two to three times a week. Start with a light weight. Slowly increase the size of your weights as your muscles become stronger.

Do stretching exercises

Stretching exercises are light or moderate physical activity. When you stretch, you increase your flexibility, lower your stress, and help prevent sore muscles.

You can choose from many types of stretching exercises. Yoga is a type of stretching that focuses on your breathing and helps you relax. Even if you have problems moving or balancing, certain types of yoga can help. For instance, chair yoga has stretches you can do when sitting in a chair or holding onto a chair while standing. Your health care team can suggest whether yoga is right for you.

2. 321 Great Tips To Successfully Manage Your Diabetes

Diabetes really is something that needs to be managed. Managing your diabetes will affect your health as you grow older. This section gives you solid advice on managing your diabetes in a way that will promote positive health and help eliminate some of the common problems those with diabetes often encounter.

1. Checking out international foods is an excellent way of finding new recipes that you'll actually enjoy eating, even though they're good for you and your Diabetes. I'd highly recommend trying Tabouleh, a Middle Eastern dish made with herbs, onions, lemon juice, and bulgur. It's extremely good mixed with hummus and served on a pita!

2. Birthday parties can be a nightmare for the parents of a diabetic child, but they don't have to be as long as you communicate with the hosts of the party. Let them know as far in the future as possible about your child's illness, and offer to

send food with them so they don't have to come up with alternatives themselves. Send enough for everyone at the party and they won't feel like they're different!

3. A Diabetic needs to take responsibility for their condition and their treatment. Therefore, it is up to you to ensure that you know absolutely everything there is to know about Diabetes. Keep up on the latest developments in medical journals so you can ask your physician for any care you think might assist you.

4. While at work, try to get in as much exercise as possible to keep your Diabetes in check. Take the stairs to the next floor to use the washroom, or go for a brisk walk around the cubicles during a break. You can even pump some iron with a bottle of water when you're on the phone!

5. Focus on leg circulation to combat diabetic Peripheral Neuropathy. Keep your feet moving as much as possible to increase the blood circulating down through your toes. One exercise that is great for a desk job is to lift your foot up and then wiggle your toes, turning your feet in circles at the ankle.

6. If you suffer from diabetes and you are going to exercise, it is important that you check your blood glucose afterward. Strenuous activity can cause your body to burn off blood glucose and if your body does not have enough glucose, you can develop hypoglycemia. If your glucose levels are too low, try eating foods that have carbs to raise your glucose levels.

7. The key to a Diabetic diet isn't necessarily cutting anything out completely, but instead is about counting up what is in that food item and eating it in an appropriate moderation. For example, having a slice of cake can be fine as long as you work it into your meal and have a smaller piece than you might have pre-diagnosis.

8. Even though your as big as a house, it's important for women with Gestational Diabetes to exercise as much as possible. Even if you're just doing yoga or going for a long walk, exercise will help you keep your weight to a reasonable level and your mind stress-free, leading to better health.

9. One of the most difficult things to remember for a newly-diagnosed diabetic is the importance of monitoring glucose levels diligently. Over time, failure to do so can lead to irreversible damage to

the nerves and blood vessels throughout the entire body. These types of damage can lead to problems with emotional, cardiovascular, and sexual health.

10. If you have diabetes, and you plan on getting pregnant or are pregnant already, it is crucial that you take extra folic acid. Babies born to a diabetic mother are more likely to develop birth defects than those born to healthy mothers and folic acid can reduce the risk of birth defects.

11. Take all of your medications that your doctor prescribes you. Follow the directions exactly, or you will not be getting the benefits of the treatment. If you have any side effects that you do not like call your doctor and they may be able to give you something else that agrees with your body better.

12. A good tip for people dealing with diabetes is to never skip meals, especially breakfast. If you do not eat for several hours for whatever reason, your body relies on glucose released from your liver for energy. People with diabetes continue to produce glucose even when their body has had enough so make sure to eat something to let your liver know to stop producing glucose.

13. Being diabetic does not mean that you must fully give up your favorite sweets, but it does mean that you must be more diligent in selecting and consuming them. To compensate for a sweet splurge, you may need to step up your exercise program, reducing your dietary intake of another sweet food, or taking more insulin.

14. Managing your blood sugar when you are a diabetic can be a challenge. Some things to keep in mind are eating the same amount at the same time everyday. This will ensure that you keep the right amount of sugar in your diet so that you can be happy and healthy.

15. Diabetes related diseases are the second largest killer in The United States. This epidemic can be avoided with daily exercise and simple changes in diet. Cut out soda, candy and fatty meats and replace them with fruit, whole grains, and lean meats. This can add years to our life.

16. When you have diabetes, there are times it may be easier to take a shot or pop a pill then to get moving. The truth is that along with a healthy diet, exercise is one of the best things you can do to take care of your body if you live with diabetes.

17. If you want to eat healthier to help overcome your Diabetes, but you just can't stomach fish without some pops of flavor on it, try capers! They're like olives in their flavor, but smaller and zestier. You can sprinkle them on any type of fish, I like to also add some slices of Spanish onion, and they take the place of sauce.

18. Diabetics need to avoid ketchup like the plague. I know it's tasty, I love it to death, but it's so full of sugar both from the tomatoes and the high fructose corn syrup that it's more of a curse than a pleasure. I like to replace it with yellow mustard as it has little to no sugar added.

19. Test your sugar regularly, and track the results. Keeping a log book of your sugar levels will help you and your doctor decide if your medication and diet plan are working to control your sugar. You can save money by sharing a glucometer with a family member or friend, so long as you do not share lancets.

20. Unless you drive a car that lacks air conditioning in super hot summer temperatures, or are on a safari in Africa, you probably don't need ice packs for your insulin. If you're worried about leaving it in the car at the mall, take it with you! I

doubt you'll have so much that it won't fit in your purse, pocket, or bag.

21. Buckwheat is an excellent choice to include in a Diabetic diet. It can lower your blood glucose levels after a meal, keeping you from having a spike. You can eat buckwheat instead of rice, or enjoy soba noodles with your dinner. It's available at almost any grocery store and is sometimes known as kasha.

22. A great breakfast food for a Diabetic is grapefruit! It's been known to assist people with weight loss even when they do nothing else. Be careful that you aren't on any pills, like atorvastatin for cholesterol, that have adverse reactions when you ingest grapefruit. It can actually increase their potency and potentially lead to an overdose.

23. To increase your sensitivity to insulin, maintain an active lifestyle. Studies have shown that insulin has a stronger effect on those who engage in plenty of physical activity. This will make sure your blood sugar levels stay in a healthy range, and will make it easier for you to manage your diabetes.

24. To keep your blood sugar levels from spiking, research high glycemic index foods. If you're not knowledgeable about what ingredients you should avoid, you may consume something harmful without realizing it. If you need to eat something quickly and don't have time to look it up, stick to non-processed foods.

25. Many people think diabetics have to avoid all sweets, but this isn't necessarily true. When planning a sweet dessert or snack, just make sure it is included in a healthy meal or with exercise. Your doctor can guide you with pointers to help you include desserts and snacks in your diet.

26. If you can't afford to get a gym membership, try your local community center or YMCA. You can find great discounts and sometimes even barter with them for a membership. For example, offer to help clean the gym or work on the grounds. That's great exercise for a diabetic, too.

27. There are ton of free ways to lose weight and battle diabetes, from jogging to doing work outs at a local park. Can goods can make inexpensive weights, as do bags filled with heavy items and chin-ups can be performed on your local park's jungle gym.

28. Eat a well-balanced diet. Since there is no official diabetes diet, it's important that you handle your condition by eating a healthy diet that is high in fruits, vegetables and lean meats and low in fat, sugar and simple carbohydrates. If you eat everything in moderation and are controlling your diabetes through medication, you should have fairly stable blood glucose levels.

29. Instead of depriving yourself of your favorite foods, look for ways to make them healthier. The difficult thing related to a diagnosis of diabetes is the way it restricts your diet. Many assume they have to stop eating these favorite foods entirely. For others, the temptations of their favorite dishes will overcome dietary restrictions. Look for alternatives to your favorite dishes if they are unhealthy. In a lot of cases, substituting healthy ingredients for diabetes-unfriendly ones can make a great dish healthier, without compromising its flavor.

30. Monitor your blood sugar at the same time every day. This helps you to know your body and to better anticipate any change of schedule or any problem. In addition, you can better control your intake of sugar, if you know what your

blood level is. Monitoring times should be as regularly as you like.

31. Something every person dealing with diabetes should know is that they can use cinnamon as a natural sweetener. Everyone understands that sugar is terrible as it can significantly affect the blood sugar level of a diabetes patient, but cinnamon offers the same sweetening effects without any risk to the patient.

32. If you are diabetic, eat high glycemic foods in moderation. This group of foods includes refined white bread, white pasta, and refined rice. These foods cause your blood sugar to raise very quickly, making it difficult to manage. Add more fruits and vegetables to your diet to avoid filling up on these processed foods.

33. Lentils are an amazing food. They are full of quality protein and nutrients. They are ideal for people with diabetes (or indeed anyone) trying to lose weight. You can do a million things with them! You can cook them and then make them into patties and eat them as hamburgers! You can sprout them in a jar and then sprinkle them in a salad! They can be found in most stores and they're not expensive - so add them to your shopping list!

34. Diabetics can have problems in their eyes due to their condition, so make sure you go to the optometrist for testing at least once a year. Many optometrists have special machines, which can look inside your eyeball to check for the typical damage of a diabetic, and can sometimes diagnose your disease before you even have symptoms!

35. Be VERY careful with any advice you receive online about diabetes treatment. It is fine to do your research online, and even to find out what other people are doing to take care of their disease, but you need to take any new information you want to act on to your doctor, to make sure that it's medically sound.

36. The best thing a person can do to avoid diabetes is to exercise. People who exercise 30 to 60 minutes per day, at least 5 days per week, can lower their risk of developing diabetes by almost 50 percent. Exercise improves the health of your heart and lungs, reduces stress, reduces fat, increases metabolism and lowers blood sugar levels.

37. If your doctor tells you that your Diabetes pills aren't doing enough to keep your blood glucose

levels in check, don't panic. You won't necessarily have to use needles as insulin pens are now available that give you the dose you need without being painful. If you can't afford these pens, some pharmaceuticals have programs to assist you like Needy Meds.

38. If you suffer from diabetes and you are going to exercise, it is important that you check your blood glucose afterward. Strenuous activity can cause your body to burn off blood glucose and if your body does not have enough glucose, you can develop hypoglycemia. If your glucose levels are too low, try eating foods that have carbs to raise your glucose levels.

39. Make sure to go to your podiatrist often if you have Diabetes to get routine foot check-ups. Your feet are susceptible to peripheral neuropathy and infection, so having them looked over will ensure you don't end up with them being amputated. It only takes a small amount of time to ensure your feet are healthy, so do it!

40. If you have a family history of heart disease, strokes or hardened arteries, you should be especially vigilant in controlling your blood glucose levels. Well-maintained levels can delay the onset of these and other medical conditions,

and can also decrease your odds of developing these diseases as you get older.

41. Here is a tip that benefits not only someone with diabetes, but anyone else. Regular exercise is important to maintain a healthy body weight, as exercise burns off excess body fat. Aerobic exercises such as jogging and cycling are good for increasing the heart rate to burn off fat.

42. Almost all insurance companies will now pay for blood glucose monitoring equipment for diabetics to have in their homes. It is important to keep machines in good working order and clean. This is vital to assure you obtain accurate results. Your manufacturer's directions have directions on how to clean and maintain your machine.

43. Be vigilant when monitoring your glucose levels. If your blood glucose levels are especially high before mealtime, this may be an indication that your liver is producing far too much glucose. Try taking your insulin 60 to 90 minutes before your meal, rather than 30 to 45 minutes beforehand. This will give your body's insulin a head start needed to more effectively manage blood glucose.

44. Although you may have little appetite and feel ill, as a diabetic you must continue to help your body by consuming healthy foods, and by tracking your blood glucose levels. If your level of glucose is low, make sure you drink plenty of water so that you do not get dehydrated.

45. To save you and your doctor time, write down all of your questions about your diabetes. This way you will be prepared ahead of time and will not forget to ask anything that is important. You are dealing with your health, so don't be afraid to ask any question that you have.

46. If you're looking to help balance your blood sugar levels, eat more whole grain foods. While no one is completely certain why it works, research indicates that whole grains are good for maintaining healthy blood sugar and also for reducing a person's risk of developing diabetes. An easy way to include more whole grains in your diet is to switch at least half the grain products you eat -- like pasta and bread -- to whole grain versions.

47. Eat a healthy diet and control your weight in order to avoid developing Type II diabetes. People who are overweight are more likely to develop diabetes, so keep your weight at an

optimal level. Eat healthy foods and limit your intake of sugar, as diabetes develops when the body is unable to process sugar properly.

48. If you're diagnosed with Diabetes or pre-Diabetes, why does the doctor prescribe exercise and lower sugar intake? It's because doing these things can often cure Diabetes! If you are exercising and eating a healthier diet, your body can process sugar better - thus lessening the ability of Diabetes to take over your life.

49. You can get a free blood glucose meter from your pharmacy just by asking. They usually have coupons or rebates so that you can get the latest model at no cost, the caveat is that you'll be buying their brand of blood test strips for the rest of your life.

50. Keep track of your blood sugar levels in a log book, so you know where you've been and how you're doing currently. If you can't afford enough test strips to check multiple times a day, check at a variety of different times, so that you can get an idea of how your sugar is going throughout a typical day.

51. Learning to read the nutrition data on food labels is key to eating the right diet for your

Diabetes. Keep track of how much carbohydrates, sodium, sugar, fat, protein, and fiber are in each food you eat and try to only choose those which will keep your weight in check.

52. When you're on a plane it can be hard for a Diabetic to keep their feet moving. Try to do little exercises while you sit, like moving your foot up and down or turning it in circles. Keep wiggling your toes to ensure your circulation gets blood right down to your tippy-toes.

53. A diet too high in protein can actually be harmful to diabetics. Some people think more protein is good, but studies have shown that too much animal protein can cause insulin-resistance, a factor in diabetes. Try to include proper amounts of protein, vegetables and carbohydrates to keep your diet healthy and well-balanced.

54. To allow yourself to still enjoy your favorite foods, make simple substitutions. Collard greens can be made with turkey broth instead of ham hock, and ground beef can easily be replaced by ground turkey. Try purchasing a diabetes cookbook. You may find that you can keep on eating many of your favorite meals.

55. Using a log book to record your daily glucose test results can be very helpful in controlling your diabetes. It is important to notice trends in your blood sugar readings, so having a written record can help you look back and see patterns. Taking a written record to your appointments can also help your doctor to make treatment adjustments.

56. It is important that you know how to use your insulin pump. Many people do not get the proper amount of insulin because they are not using their pump correctly. If you do not know what you are doing, do not feel ashamed to ask your doctor or another health professional, for help.

57. If you are the primary caregiver of a person with diabetes, you may need support also. You carry a heavy load caring for and making decisions for your loved one as well as monitoring their diet and lifestyle to keep them healthy. If you feel overwhelmed, ask for help. Your doctor can recommend respite care to give you a break, or even a nurse to help with care. You don't have to do it alone.

58. If you're trying to keep your Diabetes under control, eating right is very important. Buying fruits and vegetables in season can help you eat healthy foods while not spending more than your budget allows. Root vegetables are best to eat in winter, while berries would be cheapest in the summer months.

59. You may want to consider homeopathic medicine if you have diabetes. Some of these other natural treatments can help control symptoms just as much as medications do. For instance, Uranium nitrate helps to reduce your blood sugar while also decreasing sugar in the urine. Bryonia helps get rid of weakness and dry mouth.

60. A tip to prevent or manage diabetes is to eat high-fiber foods such as whole grains as much as possible. Processed foods, including white bread, have a high glycemic count due to being full of refined carbohydrates and these can increase the diabetes risk. This is because they lead to spikes in the blood sugar levels whereas the more natural the food, the easier it is to be digested.

61. Women, especially when in their teens and early twenties, may experience significant fluctuations in their blood glucose levels in the week

immediately leading up to their menstrual period. Monitor your levels frequently during this time, then make any necessary adjustments in your insulin dosages and urinary ketone measurements, as this can prevent further spikes.

62. You must consider fruit and high-glycemic index vegetables very carefully when planning a diet for Diabetes. Many fruits contain a LOT of sugar, which can affect your blood glucose adversely. Vegetables can cause the same problems, especially in juice form, including carrots, peas, and corn. Try to stick to low GI items like broccoli or apples which are rich in fiber.

63. Almost all insurance companies will now pay for blood glucose monitoring equipment for diabetics to have in their homes. It is important to keep machines in good working order and clean. This is vital to assure you obtain accurate results. Your manufacturer's directions have directions on how to clean and maintain your machine.

64. If you want to lower your risk for getting diabetes, you have to remain active. Try talking a fast paced walk for 60 minutes each day. When you are not focusing on working out, make sure

you are still active. Try to walk instead of drive and take the stairs instead of the elevator.

65. Clean out your pantry and fridge of all processed foods as well as foods high in sugar and trans fats. Eating trans fats and any food that has partially hydrogenated oils will increase your belly fat and put you at a higher risk for getting diabetes. These foods are not good for anyone to be eating, so it is best to toss them.

66. The number one thing to keep in mind when you're diagnosed with Type II Diabetes is that it's not the end of the world! You will be able to live a long, healthy life with this condition as long as you take the steps necessary to keep it under control.

67. Vinegar helps to keep blood sugar spikes at bay for diabetics who eat it during a meal. Some people actually recommend drinking it straight before you eat! I like to sprinkle it on a salad, or douse my vegetables in it. It's also great for marinating meats! It's extremely versatile.

68. Fish is an excellent choice of protein for a Diabetic who is looking to lose weight. It's full of Omega fatty acids which are great for your body,

and the calcium in the bones (if you include
them) can meet the daily recommended doses.

69. Stress can wreak havoc on a Diabetic's mental
health, but it will also cause problems physically
as well. Try to do stress-relieving activities like
exercise, yoga, or deep breathing exercises at the
end of the day or during any situation that is
particularly stressful to keep yourself calm, cool,
and collected.

70. Going for a walk, jog, or run with your dog, is
an excellent way to exercise and help keep your
diabetes under control. It will also help your dog
stay at a healthy weight, which can save you both
heartache and money on vet bills. You'll
motivate each other to keep going!

71. If you have Diabetes, then your children are
more susceptible to the disease themselves. Make
sure that any diet changes you make are reflected
by the eating habits of your children, and that
you include them in the exercise you do. It's
more fun to make the changes in your life if
everyone has some input.

72. Many people have diabetes. Doing this allows
ease in your life and also cuts down on the stress
and embarrassment of having diabetes.

73. A Diabetic will need more than just a physician on his health care team. You should ask for a referral to an endocrinologist (they'll help you with your insulin), a registered dietitian or nutritionist, an optometrist or ophthalmologist, a dentist, and a podiatrist. Once you have them all on your team you'll be ready to fight Diabetes head on!

74. Make sure to take your diabetes medications exactly as directed. You are NOT a doctor, nor is anyone else giving you advice other than your physician. They tell you how often to take your prescriptions and how much you should take at a time because they know, so follow their directions.

75. It is important that you eat a lot of fiber in order to prevent diabetes. Fiber helps to prevent diabetes by stabilizing your blood glucose levels. You can get fiber from certain foods such as whole grains, nuts, beans, seeds, fruits and vegetables. You can also take a fiber supplement.

76. Get familiar with the glycemic index rating of foods to help gain better control of your diabetes. It is important to learn to recognize high glycemic foods like breads, fruit juices,

cereals, pasta and rice. Eating more vegetables, lean proteins and other low glycemic index foods keeps your blood sugar from spiking after meals.

77. In addition to eating healthy foods, you should also remember to eat food regularly. Instead of eating huge meals two or three times a day like most people do, eat smaller meals spaced out through the day. Doing so will keep your blood sugar at normal levels and regulate hunger.

78. You should watch what you are eating if you have diabetes. Your blood sugar will be effected differently by various foods, so keep track of what you eat and how it will impact your blood sugar. The amount of insulin that needs to be injected depends on the size of the meals eaten. Larger meals require more insulin. If you watch what you're eating, you can manage your blood glucose levels.

79. Diabetes can affect the eyes, so make sure you are seeing an eye doctor regularly to catch any complications before they become worse. Be aware of any changes in your vision; diabetes can damage the nerves in the eyes so stay vigilant about any changes you see.

80. It is important for anyone with diabetes to check their blood sugar regularly. How often you check your blood sugar depends on your doctor's instructions, but it should be done. Checking your blood sugar allows you to see what foods raise your levels. This makes it easier to catch level spikes.

81. Understand that there is no single "magic number" when it comes to your A1C levels. However, you should aim to keep this number as low as possible in order to reduce your chances of developing complications from diabetes. Even slightly high A1C levels put you at considerable risk for stroke and cardiovascular problems.

82. If you have type 2 diabetes, and the medication you are taking is not helping as well as you had hoped, don't stress too much. Many diabetics need insulin, and they now make insulin pens that will control your blood sugar better than the syringes do. Make sure they are covered by your insurance company before getting one, because it does seem to be something insurance companies will not always approve.

83. To keep your fingertips from cracking when you check your glucose levels, clean them with an anti-bacterial soap. While using alcohol to clean

your skin may be your first instinct, it has a drying effect that makes your fingertips more susceptible to cracking. Anti-bacterial soap will ensure your hands are free of bacteria without drying them out.

84. If your doctor tells you that your Diabetes pills aren't doing enough to keep your blood glucose levels in check, don't panic. You won't necessarily have to use needles as insulin pens are now available that give you the dose you need without being painful. If you can't afford these pens, some pharmaceuticals have programs to assist you like Needy Meds.

85. If you suffer from diabetes it is absolutely critical that you monitor the amount of alcohol you drink. Cutting back on alcohol consumption is one of the best things a diabetic can do to improve their health. Alcohol is loaded with empty calories and fast acting carbohydrates. These fast acting carbohydrates quickly raise blood sugar levels in the body and this, in turn, can lead to type II diabetes complications.

86. Enroll in a diabetes class or schedule meetings with a diabetes educator. Your physician is a good source of health information, too, but an educator is specifically trained to bring medical

jargon down to your level. An educator or class can take a lot of the mystery out of your diabetes treatment plan, which is important in order for you to be active in your health care.

87. If you snore you are twice as likely to develop Diabetes than someone who doesn't. This might be because most people who snore are overweight, and it's the extra weight that can lead to Diabetes. Deal with the weight and you'll conquer both the snoring and the Diabetes!

88. Eat foods rich in fiber. By eating fruits, vegetables, and grains you will improve your diet. You will lose weight and feel great. Fiber can help give you more control over your blood sugar and lower your chances of getting heart disease. Other sources of fiber include nuts, seeds, and beans.

89. A diet too high in protein can actually be harmful to diabetics. Some people think more protein is good, but studies have shown that too much animal protein can cause insulin-resistance, a factor in diabetes. Try to include proper amounts of protein, vegetables and carbohydrates to keep your diet healthy and well-balanced.

90. A great way to save money and still eat healthy is to plan out all your meals. If you can reuse a food bought in bulk multiple times, like a loaf of bread or a specific vegetable, you'll be able to save money on the purchase. Plan out every meal to make the most of your grocery buys.

91. Anyone with diabetes must exercise to stay in good health. Exercise helps strengthen the cardiovascular system and helps to increase the circulation to the arms and legs. It also helps to control blood sugar levels. The best forms of exercise for someone with diabetes is jogging, swimming, walking, and rowing.

92. To sate your sweet tooth without putting your health at risk, cut any unnecessary carbohydrates from your diet. Reducing your carbohydrate intake can be enough to make a small cookie or a slice of pie okay. Talk to your doctor about your diet and see how many carbohydrates you'd have to cut in order to enjoy your favorite sweets.

93. If you suffer from Diabetes, a helpful tip is to eat bars or shakes especially made for Diabetics in between your meals when you are out. Doing this can keep your glucose levels even. However, you want to avoid having these in addition to your meals because that will cause your glucose

levels to climb. Only use them as meal replacements!

94. Many diabetics feel harassed by loved ones who are always inquiring about their blood sugars and testing habits. Instead of becoming frustrated or resentful, sit down with the other person and clearly identify what steps they can take in order to more effectively contribute to managing your condition. Chances are, the other person is not trying to irritate you, but instead is looking for ways to help out.

95. Due to the nature of diabetes and the circulation issues it can cause, you need to always pay attention to your feet and make sure that there are no infections developing. This is important because it is very easy to get an infection that could lead to the need for amputation if not caught in time or severe blood poisoning from dying skin tissue.

96. One of the best methods for the prevention of diabetes is a healthy lifestyle. Although it can be genetic, there are other factors, such as nutrition and weight, which contribute to diabetes. Staying active and keeping a well-balanced diet will lower your risk of developing diabetes in the future.

97. There is really no need to swab your skin with an alcohol swab before you give yourself an injection. The alcohol is going to dry your skin out and that could cause the injections to be more painful. If you are prone to infections, you may want to continue to swab before the injection to prevent infection.

98. Get enough sleep. Poor sleep habits or simply not getting enough sleep can impact many aspects of your health, including your diabetes. Studies have shown that even one night of lost sleep can cause a 25 percent decrease in insulin sensitivity. Losing sleep can also cause your hormones to become unstable, which often leads to an increased appetite and consequently a higher glucose level.

99. When it comes to dealing with diabetes, one important point to consider is that you should look into having your medications sent to your home instead of going out to pick them up. This will be a great advantage for you because you can save time and gas money.

100.   If you have type II Diabetes then it's time to say goodbye to fried foods. The breading on most fried food is full of carbohydrates, typically has sugar added to it, and soaks up unhealthy

oils. You really don't want to be ingesting any of these unhealthy things.

101.   For people with diabetes, it is important to check your glucose level after heavy exercise. Exercise can keep consuming glucose for up to 24 hours later, so it's best to check your glucose level every 45 minutes or so after your workout to see if your glucose level is dropping or remaining stable.

102.   Quit smoking. Try again if you've tried before. Nicotine constricts your blood vessels. Diabetes already have a problem with circulation to the extremeties; that's what leads to vision problems and the need for amputations. Smoking increases these risks, as well as being bad for your health overall. Ask your doctor for some resources to help you quit.

103.   Diabetics should beware of caffeine as it can lead to potentially life-threatening blood pressure. Diabetes already has harmful effects on your organs, high blood pressure included, so you don't want to tax your body any more than it already is. Caffeine can lead in a massive spike in blood pressure after ingesting it, so just stay away from it completely.

104.   A Diabetic will need more than just a physician on his health care team. You should ask for a referral to an endocrinologist (they'll help you with your insulin), a registered dietitian or nutritionist, an optometrist or ophthalmologist, a dentist, and a podiatrist. Once you have them all on your team you'll be ready to fight Diabetes head on!

105.   You can find the most common Diabetic supplies and medications available at some grocery stores for a significant discount. This can help you keep your medical bills in check, leading you to be more likely to take your medications as instructed. Feel free to reuse your syringes a few times, that will also save you money.

106.   To allow yourself to still enjoy your favorite foods, make simple substitutions. Collard greens can be made with turkey broth instead of ham hock, and ground beef can easily be replaced by ground turkey. Try purchasing a diabetes cookbook. You may find that you can keep on eating many of your favorite meals.

107.   To keep your diabetes from hurting your teeth, be sure to brush and floss several times a day. Diabetes increases the levels of glucose in your saliva, which means your teeth are much

more susceptible to decay. Anyone suffering from diabetes needs to be extra vigilante when it comes to taking care of their teeth.

108.   Even if you "only" have Gestational Diabetes, it is especially important for you to monitor your blood glucose levels. Your baby will be impacted by the slightest peak you might have as the insulin does cross the placenta, so make sure to keep your levels even so your baby will grow normally.

109.   At every grocery store you walk into today, you will be able to find bars or shakes that are for diabetics. If you find that you are having trouble controlling your blood glucose levels when you are out and about, carry these with you at all times for an easy and safe meal on the go.

110.   Stop smoking. Aside from the well-documented lung cancer risks, smoking is of extra concern for diabetics. Diabetes and smoking both put you at an increased risk for heart disease, nerve damage, and kidney problems. Smoking also causes a rise in blood sugar. Either risk alone is enough for concern, but a diabetic who smokes is at a much higher risk of developing problems.

111.   People suffering from Diabetes should consider adding green tea to their diet as a replacement of other sugary drinks. Green tea is a great way to cut calories and save carbohydrates. It also has the added benefit of fighting several other diseases. It may not lower your blood sugar, but it helps in many other ways.

112.   To maintain healthy blood sugar levels, maintain a healthy, regular routine. That is, try to eat around the same amount of food daily and eat at the same times, and also exercise and take medications at the same times of day. In combination with healthy practices, spacing things out like this helps keep your blood sugar on an even keel throughout the day.

113.   Insulin is being developed that can be inhaled. This will prove to be a great alternative to injections that many diabetics are forced to endure. Meanwhile this product is still undergoing clinical trials, it is said to be available within the United States and Europe within as little as a few years. Consider this in the near future for a positive alternative to insulin injections.

114.   The food you eat is not the only thing that affects your blood glucose level. To help decrease your glucose level, you should make sure you spend a little bit of time each day doing some exercise. When you exercise, your body uses glucose and it could burn the glucose even if you exercised 24 hours ago.

115.   Control when and how much you eat. Try to eat meals and snacks at the same time every day. Eating at the same time will keep your blood sugar regulated and make it easier to maintain. How much you eat is important because even if you eat healthy, but overeat, you can gain weight.

116.   The number one thing to keep in mind when you're diagnosed with Type II Diabetes is that it's not the end of the world! You will be able to live a long, healthy life with this condition as long as you take the steps necessary to keep it under control.

117.   If you don't like the taste of beans but are trying to eat properly now that you've been diagnosed with Diabetes, why not try eating Hummus? It is made from creamed Garbanzo Beans and it's smooth, thick, and delicious! You can eat it on a sandwich instead of mayonnaise, or spread on crackers.

118.   If you want to eat healthier to help overcome your Diabetes, but you just can't stomach fish without some pops of flavor on it, try capers! They're like olives in their flavor, but smaller and zestier. You can sprinkle them on any type of fish, I like to also add some slices of Spanish onion, and they take the place of sauce.

119.   If you want a fun way to exercise, take your kids to the park! You can play a game of soccer or basketball, or just chase them around on the playground. Tennis is also fun and you can play with kids of any age. Pick something they enjoy and you'll enjoy it, too!

120.   Eating fresh, non-processed foods is an easy way for a diabetic to keep his or her weight in check and blood sugar stable. By shopping only the outside aisles of the grocery store you will find you're not exposed to the processed sugary or carbohydrate-laden treats, that can lead to temptation.

121.   If you have a family history of diabetes, prevention is very important. A great way to prevent diabetes is to increase your intake of fiber. Foods that are high in fiber include fruits, vegetables, beans, whole grains and nuts. Foods

high in fiber increase your blood sugar control ability, which in turn reduces your chances of getting diabetes. Filling your plate up with foods high in fiber is an important way to prevent diabetes.

122.   Do not eat snacks out of a bag. By eating snacks directly from its container, you are more likely to overeat and create a spike in your blood sugar levels. Get a plate and put a small portion on the plate. Eat it slowly, savor the flavor, and don't get more after you have finished.

123.   It is important that you have your cholesterol checked at least once a year if you have diabetes. Having diabetes increases your chances of developing high cholesterol, which can cause serious health problems like heart disease and stroke. There is a simple blood test called a fasting lipid profile that checks your cholesterol levels.

124.   To keep your diabetes from hurting your teeth, be sure to brush and floss several times a day. Diabetes increases the levels of glucose in your saliva, which means your teeth are much more susceptible to decay. Anyone suffering from diabetes needs to be extra vigilante when it comes to taking care of their teeth.

125.   Educate yourself. Being diagnosed with diabetes can be a scary prospect, so seek out information in order to be prepared and know what to expect. You can look into a class at your local community college, or check with the American Diabetes Association, as they have a team of educators who hold informational meetings you can attend.

126.   When you have diabetes, there are several ways that you can reduce your consumption of sugar. Instead of a sugar-laden soft drink, drink a serving of sparkling water. Substitute a bowl of frozen fruit for a bowl of strawberry ice cream. Instead of a slice of cake, enjoy a slice of cheese. Substitute a wedge of apple for a serving of apple pie.

127.   When dealing with a child that has diabetes, be sure to not let that be an excuse for your child to not participate in activities that he or she would have normally done, otherwise. This is crucial because despite having this disease, children cannot be deprived of their childhood. This includes activities, such as, participating in sports or play dates with other children.

128.   For effective diabetes control through diet, regulate the amount of food you eat. Avoiding overeating keeps your blood sugar from skyrocketing and causing problems, because the amount of food you eat affects how much sugar is in your blood. Don't eat too little, either, though, because that kind of imbalance can also cause illness.

129.   To maintain healthy blood sugar levels, maintain a healthy, regular routine. That is, try to eat around the same amount of food daily and eat at the same times, and also exercise and take medications at the same times of day. In combination with healthy practices, spacing things out like this helps keep your blood sugar on an even keel throughout the day.

130.   Afraid of diabetes? Its time to start exercising. Not only will we get that body that we always wanted if we exercise, but also we will lessen our chance of getting diabetes. Every calorie we burn on that treadmill can add time to our life. If you are looking for reasons to exercise think of how much you can extend your life by dedicating that 30 minutes everyday.

131.   It is OK to give into temptation every once in a while. No one is perfect and to keep you

from feeling like you are missing out on life too much, you should let yourself have a little bit. Just be sure that it does not become too much of a habit.

132.   Hey there, Diabetics! Have you ever thought of turning your burger inside out? Well, not exactly, but putting the lettuce on the outside will get rid of that carbohydrate-laced bun and increase the amount of vegetables you're eating. Replace the hamburger with a lentil patty for an even healthier treat!

133.   Skip the french fries and ditch the baked potato - it's time to replace your carb-heavy side dishes with something that's actually GOOD for a Diabetic. Salad! I'm not talking potato or pasta salad, they're both carbohydrate disaster areas. Pick up some lettuce, shred some vegetables, throw on some tomato wedges and a nice light oil and vinegar dressing and dig in!

134.   Diabetics MUST visit their doctor regularly to keep tabs on their blood sugar, weight, and medications. Your physician might know of a new treatment that could be useful to you, or see something in your blood work that indicates there is a problem. Having your doctor weigh you will also give you an accurate measurement

of how well you're keeping your weight under
control.

135.   Herbal tea is a great drink for diabetics as it
contains many wonderful nutrients and can taste
so good you don't even think about adding
cream or sugar. Be sure to check the ingredients
as some manufacturers will add sugar or artificial
sweeteners.

136.   Lower the risk of getting diabetes by eating a
diet high in fiber. Whole grains are low-GI
foods, which reduces your risk of diabetes, while
white foods are generally high-GI, which
increases your risk. Research demonstrates that
diets rich in whole grain are at lesser risk of
suffering diabetes.

137.   Be passionate about having Diabetes and
become an advocate for the disease. Type II
Diabetes is preventable, and it's costing our
government billions of dollars in treatment for
people who can't afford it. You may not be one
of those who are tapping the system for your
care, but speaking up about what you know to
help others avoid the disease will help us be able
to use our money for more important things.

138.   Try buying food at local farmer's markets or at the farm itself to get discounts on healthy foods. A diet for Diabetes doesn't have to be expensive, you just have to look for deals and sometimes shop in different locations. Eating farm fresh eggs for the first time will make you a believer!

139.   If you're diabetic, beware coupons! Most coupons to be found, are often, for items that aren't healthy, like pop, crackers or chips. Do not use a coupon just because you have it! You might save 50 cents today, but the cost of medications to deal with an obesity-related illness later, will add up to much more.

140.   Make sure to go to your podiatrist often if you have Diabetes to get routine foot check-ups. Your feet are susceptible to peripheral neuropathy and infection, so having them looked over will ensure you don't end up with them being amputated. It only takes a small amount of time to ensure your feet are healthy, so do it!

141.   To make sure you don't suffer from diabetes-related complications, always get plenty of sleep. Studies have show that people suffering from sleep deprivation eat much more food, which will make it difficult to keep your diabetes

under control. A good night's rest will also help your body to keep your blood sugar levels in check.

142.   Paper and pen are your greatest weapons in defeating Diabetes. You should keep track of your exercise via a log, a diet diary to see what causes you blood-glucose spikes, blood pressure log, blood sugar reading log, and when you take your medications and how much, you have taken.

143.   If you're feeling burned out by your diabetes care don't brush your feelings aside! Ignoring your emotions can lead to you slipping in your care, which can in turn lead to more serious health problems. If you're stressed it will also be more difficult to keep your blood sugar levels stable. Talk to your doctor when you're feeling overwhelmed, and work together to find a way to simplify your diabetes management.

144.   Remove contributors to the complications of diabetes. Try to avoid unhealthy habits that will affect your heart health and chances for stroke. Smoking should be stopped at all costs, maintain a healthy blood pressure through stress management and salt control and evaluate

lifestyle choices that can have less than favorable results.

145.   If you are a diabetic who has never smoked, or who has not smoked in 6 months, you may want to talk with your doctor about using an inhaled insulin treatment. Recent medical studies have shown that inhaled insulin may be more effective in treating diabetes than pills or injections.

146.   A good tip for people dealing with diabetes is to never skip meals, especially breakfast. If you do not eat for several hours for whatever reason, your body relies on glucose released from your liver for energy. People with diabetes continue to produce glucose even when their body has had enough so make sure to eat something to let your liver know to stop producing glucose.

147.   To avoid sugar but still sweeten your food, ask about neotame. Neotame is an FDA approved sweetener that has been confirmed safe for sufferers of diabetes. Neotame is extremely sweet, so only a small amount needs to be used. This will allow you to curb your sweet tooth without jeopardizing your health.

148.   Thintini buns are available at many grocery stores nation-wide and are a tasty alternative to carbohydrate-heavy normal hamburger buns. These thinner breads are easier to eat as they're smaller than their traditional counterparts and they will provide far less carbohydrates to a diabetic.

149.   If you feel you're not getting adequate care from your doctor, find a new one! Feeling less than comfortable with a health care professional can lead you to question their diagnosis or treatment, meaning you can't trust them. Find a new doctor that you have full faith in to ensure a healthy doctor-patient relationship.

150.   A Diabetic needs to have eight good hours of sleep every night to be well-rested, alert, and healthy. People who get enough sleep tend to be able to lose weight, probably because they have the energy to exercise and lack the apathy that can lead to less than healthy eating choices.

151.   Enroll in a diabetes class or schedule meetings with a diabetes educator. Your physician is a good source of health information, too, but an educator is specifically trained to bring medical jargon down to your level. An educator or class can take a lot of the mystery

out of your diabetes treatment plan, which is important in order for you to be active in your health care.

152.   If you want to add a nutritious touch to your salad, throw in some walnuts! Walnuts contain monounsaturated fats. These fats are great at helping to control diabetes. In addition, they contain antioxidants, minerals, omega-3s and vitamins. They also boost your energy and taste delicious!

153.   If you have been diagnosed with Diabetes - keep a diet diary! This is a handy tool! A diary will allow you to track what and how much you are eating. It will also help you detect a pattern you may have for a certain craving at a particular time of the day. You will be able to see which foods cause your blood glucose level to spike. Perhaps you can make some tasty alternatives that will not have such an effect on your Diabetes? Doing so will help you to avoid any unnecessary headaches.

154.   If you're trying to keep your Diabetes under control, eating right is very important. Buying fruits and vegetables in season can help you eat healthy foods while not spending more than your budget allows. Root vegetables are best to eat in

winter, while berries would be cheapest in the summer months.

155.   Eating out at restaurants or getting take out is not only bad for a Diabetic's health, but also their checkbook. Save money and your blood glucose level by eating at home instead. You can find many copycat recipes online for all your favorite foods, and even healthier versions which are better for you.

156.   Even if you feel like your diabetes has gotten better, it is important not to stop taking your medications unless a doctor tells you it is alright to do so. The medications are most likely what is keeping your diabetes symptoms under control, so without them, your glucose or insulin levels could get out of control.

157.   Live a fun life. Don't let diabetes get you down. You may have to watch your blood glucose levels, but you can still lead a full, enjoyable life. Have hobbies, to out with friends and even eat at a restaurant. Diabetes is a condition you have, but it isn't you.

158.   Be careful to not rely on diabetes candy bars and shakes too often. Although they are good for people on the go, they do not replace eating a

meal. If you end up eating the candy bars or drinking the shakes too much, you could actually cause your blood glucose level to go too high.

159.   Try drinking green tea if you suffer from diabetes. It is a great way to give into your sweet tooth without drinking a beverage that could affect your blood sugar. Also, although nothing has been proven, doctors are looking into the suggestion that green tea may actually lower blood sugar.

160.   To make sure you choose the right carbohydrates, avoid white foods. White bread, pasta, or rice are all made from refined carbohydrates, which means they are also high glycemic index foods. Getting your carbohydrates from whole wheat products will ensure that your glucose levels stay stable, and that your body is able to digest them properly.

161.   When it comes to dealing with diabetes, be sure that you keep a journal with your blood sugar levels on a regular basis. This is important to stay on top of in order to reduce the risk of stroke, heart disease, and other potentially fatal side effects. Keeping a journal will help to identify why you might have low or high levels at a certain time.

162.   With diabetes, it is important that you consult with professional help right away. This is important because there is plenty to be learned about the disease that only someone who specializes in it will know. Other than paid doctor visits, there are also toll free numbers that you can call for guidance.

163.   To reduce the risk of heart disease associated with diabetes, watch your fat intake. Avoiding unhealthy fats like saturated fats and trans fats is even more important for diabetics than for other people because of their association with heart disease. Replacing bad fats with good fats like olive oil is better for your overall health. Also, watch the amount of fats you eat, since weight control is an important part of diabetes control.

164.   Check the glycemic index to determine how much different foods will affect your blood sugar level. Select foods with a low glycemic index.

165.   If you're having trouble getting the motivation to exercise after being diagnosed with Type II Diabetes, get in the game! Competitive sports are not only fun, but you have other people who rely on you to show up so that there are enough players for a game. Having them

breathing down your neck will convince you to be on time!

166.   Be careful with the medicines you choose when you have a cold, many are laden with sugar which can affect your blood sugar levels. Make sure you take this into account if you're keeping track of what you eat to maintain even blood sugar levels, or if your blood sugar mysteriously spikes.

167.   If you are diabetic, be sure to wear loose-fitting socks and stockings. Special socks are available for diabetics that have more stretch around the ankles and legs, to provide better comfort and circulation, as well as, to help keep your feet and legs healthier. Good circulation is imperative for the legs and feet of diabetics.

168.   Be passionate about having Diabetes and become an advocate for the disease. Type II Diabetes is preventable, and it's costing our government billions of dollars in treatment for people who can't afford it. You may not be one of those who are tapping the system for your care, but speaking up about what you know to help others avoid the disease will help us be able to use our money for more important things.

169.   If you have diabetes, it is important that you take care of your feet. Simple cuts can turn into infections for diabetics, which in turn can cause serious health problems, such as gangrene and even amputation. Check your feet daily and if you notice any cuts or other irregularities, see your doctor.

170.   Baking your own bread, canning your own vegetables, and even grinding your own flour is far more healthy than purchasing it at a store. You'll also save a ton of money, and you'll know what is going into the foods you eat. A diabetic has to be careful about every ingredient, and if YOU measured and put them all in there, it will make keeping track easy!

171.   To keep stress from elevating your blood sugar, try practicing meditation. Meditation is a quick and easy way to calm yourself down and keep your blood sugar levels stable. If you're feeling irritable or overwhelmed, excuse yourself, sit down, and take a few minutes to meditate. It'll make your diabetes much easier to manage.

172.   Being diagnosed with Type II Diabetes does not mean you are lazy, fat, or nonathletic. There are many causes of Diabetes which don't necessarily come from being overweight or not

exercising enough, but all diagnoses mean that you'll need to start watching what you're eating and increase your exercise level.

173.   A Diabetic diet can include many "bad" foods as long as you reduce your portions. MANY studies have shown that people who live to a hundred eat a diet that is very restrictive on calories. This leads them to have healthy organs, strong minds, and a long, happy, vigorous life.

174.   If you are feeling symptoms of depression, consult with your physician. If you become depressed it will have a severe impact on how you are managing your diabetes. You will lose interest in food, have a lower activity level and increase your stress levels. Targeting these symptoms early can avoid unwanted complications later.

175.   Be vigilant when monitoring your glucose levels. If your blood glucose levels are especially high before mealtime, this may be an indication that your liver is producing far too much glucose. Try taking your insulin 60 to 90 minutes before your meal, rather than 30 to 45 minutes beforehand. This will give your body's insulin a head start needed to more effectively manage blood glucose.

176.   Diabetics are much more prone to gum disease, therefore proper mouth care is vital. Careful brushing and flossing of the teeth are a necessity and frequent dental visits may be needed. Avoid dentures that are ill fitting and may cause mouth sores. Follow these tips for a healthy dental check up if you have diabetes.

177.   If you are a diabetic, consider seeking the help of a nutritionist. A nutritionist is able to help you with problems as such as: what to eat, what you can't eat, what diets to follow and what to eat as a bedtime snack. Nutritionists also provide assistance in answering questions you may have.

178.   It is OK to give into temptation every once in a while. No one is perfect and to keep you from feeling like you are missing out on life too much, you should let yourself have a little bit. Just be sure that it does not become too much of a habit.

179.   Make sure you pack your snacks to control your blood sugar. Good snacks include raisins, fruit juice, or hard sweets like toffees or mints. Quick access to these type of snacks can make a

world of difference in controlling your blood sugar.

180.   Make an effort to slim down if you have diabetes. Even just a few pounds makes a big difference when it comes to how your body uses insulin. Less weight means lower blood sugar and blood pressure. You will also feel more energized. An easy way to begin is by reducing the amount of calories you eat from fatty foods, like chips.

181.   Beans for breakfast, beans for tea, beans for you and beans for me! Beans are packed full of protein and fiber, which are both very important in the meals of a diabetic. Try to include as many beans and lentils in the foods you eat as possible. Just cook them up and throw them into everything, from chili to salads!

182.   If your child is diagnosed with type 1 diabetes, you might think your life is ruined, but it isn't. The treatment of diabetes has advanced tremendously in the last few years, and your child can have a normal life if they take care of themselves properly. The world's oldest living diabetic has lived for 90 years and has been around since before the current medical advances.

183.   Stress can wreak havoc on a Diabetic's mental health, but it will also cause problems physically as well. Try to do stress-relieving activities like exercise, yoga, or deep breathing exercises at the end of the day or during any situation that is particularly stressful to keep yourself calm, cool, and collected.

184.   It's not something that you should feel ashamed about, especially since it's increasingly common. Doing this allows ease in your life and also cuts down on the stress and embarrassment of having diabetes.

185.   Don't use alcohol swabs before an insulin injection. It's actually unnecessary, as long as your skin, hands, and needle are clean. Alcohol swabs will dry out the skin, making it more likely that the injection site will stay open. This can actually increase the risk of an infection at the site.

186.   In addition to eating healthy foods, you should also remember to eat food regularly. Instead of eating huge meals two or three times a day like most people do, eat smaller meals spaced out through the day. Doing so will keep your blood sugar at normal levels and regulate hunger.

187.   If you feel that your medication is not working to control your diabetes, you may want to talk to your doctor about switching medications. There are a wide variety of different diabetic medications and what works for one person, may not work well for you. Or your dosage may need to be increased.

188.   If you have diabetes and you smoke, try to stop. Smoking is bad for your health generally, but it is especially dangerous for those with diabetes because it can spike your glucose levels dangerously high. If you are finding it difficult to quit smoking, your doctor may be able to offer some help.

189.   To assist your body in digesting your good properly, be sure to chew your food slowly. When you chew your food, it's covered in enzymes that help your body to process what you eat. Doing this will make sure your body is able to take equal advantage of all the nutrients you consume, keeping your glucose levels stable.

190.   By way of advice one of the best suggestions for a diabetic is to know themselves. You know better than anybody how your body will react to that small ice cream, or how low your blood

sugars will get if you wait to long for your meal. Know yourself, and use that knowledge to more effectively manage your diabetes.

191.   It is crucial that people with diabetes get a simple blood test known as an HbA1c test every three months. HbA1c tests show blood sugar levels for the past two to three months and can help your doctor control your diabetes. It is recommended that the HbA1c is kept at or below seven percent.

192.   Do not rely solely upon urine ketone testing to measure your blood glucose levels. You should also make sure you know what the normal range is at various times during the day. Instead of this method, it is recommended by the ADA to use testing strips and finger pricks, which are more accurate.

193.   Prospective employers are forbidden from barring applicants from employment based upon a diagnosis of diabetes. You have a right to privacy and do not have to tell them about your diabetes.

194.   Try strength training. Most people are aware that exercise is beneficial for everybody, and especially for diabetics. However, often the

emphasis is put on cardiovascular exercises. These stamina-building aerobic activities are an important part of a good exercise regime, but don't forget to include some strength training. Strength training has been shown to reduce the amount of fat found inside the body cavity, surrounding your organs making it just as heart-healthy as traditional cardiovascular exercises.

195.   Do not skip any meals if you are a diabetic. Doing that will cause you to be more hungry when it is time to eat and you will probably eat much more than you would have otherwise. This will lead to higher than usual blood sugar levels so it should be avoided.

196.   When you have diabetes, it is important that you remain as active as possible. This is important to keep your overall immune system in as good as shape as possible as well as ensuring that you have a healthy circulation system. Park the car in a further away parking spot or take the stairs when they are an option.

197.   It is beneficial to keep a blood glucose monitoring system in your home if you are a diabetic. Most insurance companies will pay for your blood glucose monitoring system. To receive accurate results, make sure that you keep

your equipment clean and in a safe environment. Doing so will ensure your results are accurate and your equipment lasts for a long time.

198.   The number one thing to keep in mind when you're diagnosed with Type II Diabetes is that it's not the end of the world! You will be able to live a long, healthy life with this condition as long as you take the steps necessary to keep it under control.

199.   Keep track of all the medicines you are taking for your Diabetes and any other condition you have in case you ever need to know. You should carry with you information on their names, dosages, and how often you are taking them in case something happens to you when you're out, or a doctor you're visiting requests that information.

200.   If you are diabetic, one of the most important tips to follow is to have a proper diet. A proper diet consists of plenty of fruits, vegetables, lean protein, whole grains and low-fat dairy products. This type of diet is important for overall health for anybody, but for diabetics it's important in order to keep blood sugar under control. As an added benefit, following a diet plan like this will also help you to lose weight.

201.   If you have a family history of diabetes, prevention is very important. A great way to prevent diabetes is to increase your intake of fiber. Foods that are high in fiber include fruits, vegetables, beans, whole grains and nuts. Foods high in fiber increase your blood sugar control ability, which in turn reduces your chances of getting diabetes. Filling your plate up with foods high in fiber is an important way to prevent diabetes.

202.   DefeatDiabetes.org helps people who are struggling financially to receive supplies which will help them keep their diabetes under control. You can get as much as 35% cash back on purchases through their store, and they have additional programs to give you even deeper discounts if you ask for help through their website.

203.   Diabetics can help to avoid drastic changes in post-workout glucose levels by taking added steps to monitor their levels, as often as 45 minutes following a particularly rigorous exercise routine. Because glucose levels can continue to drop for an entire day after workouts, this will keep you from being caught unaware.

204.   Find out if there are any public gardening areas near you where people grow their own produce. This is an excellent way for a Diabetic to get some exercise by doing weeding, watering, or planting new seedlings. Often you get to keep some of what you grow as well, giving you some wonderfully fresh and organic treats to enjoy when you get home!

205.   Following the USDA Food Guide Pyramid will help you to live healthier with diabetes. The food guide pyramid was developed as a guide for healthy eating for everyone. It works for people with diabetes, too. The shape of the pyramid tells you how much to eat of different foods.

206.   To better control your blood sugars, lose any excess weight. If you're suffering from type 2 diabetes even a small decrease in weight can significantly improve your condition. Try eating more non-processed foods and reducing your portion sizes. You can also try getting a moderate amount of aerobic exercises. All these things will help you manage your diabetes as you lose weight.

207.   If you are diagnosed as a diabetic it may be in your best interests to carry around a glucose gel. You simply never know when your blood

sugars will jump, and consequently, when you might need a quick rush of sugar to your body. Keeping it handy can and will save your life.

208.   Cut down on simple carbohydrates. These foods, such as pasta and bread, cause your blood sugar levels to spike which may cause hyperglycemia and a need for more insulin; that may result in a hypoglycemic episode. Stick to complex carbohydrates such as whole grains in order to keep your blood sugar stable.

209.   Make sure that if you are diabetic and you are going to be traveling by airplane, that you drink a lot of water. The cabin's air is a lot drier than normal air is and it can cause thirst, especially in those that have diabetes. You should be able to pass through airport security with water bottles if you can prove that you have diabetes.

210.   If you are planning to travel via plane, take additional precautions to protect your insulin during the trip. If your insulin is in a piece of luggage that is checked, you risk that it is exposed to especially hot or cold, even freezing, temperatures. Always keep it with you when you fly.

211.   Eating sugar is a big no-no when you have diabetes. So, you should try to use a sugar substitute for anything that you would normally use sugar for. You can also use honey because it is a natural form of sugar, and the body will break it down much easier.

212.   Before going to a restaurant for dinner you should have a piece of fruit or a few veggie sticks. This will prevent you from going to a restaurant and nibbling on the bread basket or chips that restaurants usually give patrons while they are waiting on their meals to be prepared.

213.   Diabetes does not have to keep one from doing the things that they wish to do and enjoy. By properly monitoring ones blood sugar and doing the necessary things to maintain it one can enjoy their life still. One can have an excellent quality of life regardless of their diabetes.

214.   Keep track of your blood sugar levels in a log book, so you know where you've been and how you're doing currently. If you can't afford enough test strips to check multiple times a day, check at a variety of different times, so that you can get an idea of how your sugar is going throughout a typical day.

215.   To increase your sensitivity to insulin, maintain an active lifestyle. Studies have shown that insulin has a stronger effect on those who engage in plenty of physical activity. This will make sure your blood sugar levels stay in a healthy range, and will make it easier for you to manage your diabetes.

216.   It is important that you have your cholesterol checked at least once a year if you have diabetes. Having diabetes increases your chances of developing high cholesterol, which can cause serious health problems like heart disease and stroke. There is a simple blood test called a fasting lipid profile that checks your cholesterol levels.

217.   Baking your own bread, canning your own vegetables, and even grinding your own flour is far more healthy than purchasing it at a store. You'll also save a ton of money, and you'll know what is going into the foods you eat. A diabetic has to be careful about every ingredient, and if YOU measured and put them all in there, it will make keeping track easy!

218.   Eat a well-balanced diet. Since there is no official diabetes diet, it's important that you handle your condition by eating a healthy diet

that is high in fruits, vegetables and lean meats and low in fat, sugar and simple carbohydrates. If you eat everything in moderation and are controlling your diabetes through medication, you should have fairly stable blood glucose levels.

219.   If you have diabetes, you want to make sure you limit the amount of pasta you consume. It is really easy to eat too much of it because it is so delicious. Before you know it, you will eat more than you think you have eaten, which can really elevate your glucose levels. A cup of pasta has as many calories as three slices of bread. Keep that in mind the next time you eat pasta.

220.   If you suffer from diabetes and you are on Metformin, beware of lactic acidosis. This is a rare, but deadly condition that occurs when lactic acid develops in the bloodstream faster than in can be removed. This is more common in older people who take Metofrmin and symptoms include extreme weakness and severe nausea.

221.   If you're feeling burned out by your diabetes care don't brush your feelings aside! Ignoring your emotions can lead to you slipping in your care, which can in turn lead to more serious health problems. If you're stressed it will also be

more difficult to keep your blood sugar levels stable. Talk to your doctor when you're feeling overwhelmed, and work together to find a way to simplify your diabetes management.

222.   When you have diabetes, there are several ways that you can reduce your consumption of sugar. Instead of a sugar-laden soft drink, drink a serving of sparkling water. Substitute a bowl of frozen fruit for a bowl of strawberry ice cream. Instead of a slice of cake, enjoy a slice of cheese. Substitute a wedge of apple for a serving of apple pie.

223.   People with diabetes are at a higher risk of developing heart disease than others so they should try to eat food that contain fatty acids, which are very good for the heart. A good way to get those essential acids in your system is to have fish at least twice a week.

224.   Even though carbohydrates have a huge impact on a person's blood sugar levels, a person who has diabetes does not have to totally avoid them. However, you should be wise about what types of carbohydrates you consume. Complex carbohydrates, such as those found in whole grain brown rice and rolled oats, cause you to stay full longer since they digest slowly. They also

aid in keeping your blood sugar level more stable.

225.   If you are a diabetic seeking exercise, make sure that you stay away from any exercises that require the weight lifting and pushing or pulling heavy objects. During this kind of exercise, blood pressure and blood sugar levels are raised which can lead to many harmful health factors. To be on the safe side, avoid such exercises and keep your lifting to a minimum.

226.   If someone is still new to diabetes, it is essential that he or she quickly learn as much as he or she can about this condition. Education is key so that diabetes patients know exactly how to take proper care of themselves and keep their condition well-managed. Information and continuous learning give a diabetic power to responsibly take steps toward staying as healthy as possible.

227.   When you are testing your blood glucose levels, take the time to wash your hands properly before you perform the test on yourself. Use an antibacterial soap that is mild in nature so that you keep your fingertips moist. This will make the test much more effective and your hands more moisturized.

228. Keep your stress levels low. Diabetics can often experience an increase in glucose levels during times of stress. Try yoga or meditation to relax yourself and keep your glucose levels in check. In addition, there are a number of breathing exercises that you can teach yourself. Since you can do them anywhere, they are ideal.

229. For people with diabetes, it is important to check your glucose level after heavy exercise. Exercise can keep consuming glucose for up to 24 hours later, so it's best to check your glucose level every 45 minutes or so after your workout to see if your glucose level is dropping or remaining stable.

230. Diabetics should never EVER skip a meal! If you've planned to eat, then you must eat, or else your medication can drop your blood sugar so low you end up getting very sick. At least have a drink of juice or milk and some of your food so that your body gets a boost of energy.

231. The more you exercise, the more insulin sensitive you become. Even if you're not feeling well or injured you'll need to find something to do that gets your heart pumping. If your legs aren't working, use your arms, or vice versa.

Even rolling around on the floor can get your Diabetes in check.

232.   In order to be healthy in the midst of having diabetes, it is very important to eat the right kind of food. It is good to switch to food that is high in fiber such as whole grains. These types of foods contain refined carbohydrates that help decrease the risks associated with diabetes.

233.   People who eat at least two servings of dairy a day are less likely to develop insulin resistance, even if they're significantly over weight. Even if you're already Diabetic, including lots of low-fat dairy in your diet will help you to keep your blood sugar levels under control all day.

234.   If you have diabetes or are at risk for developing it, it is important that you lose weight. Being overweight or obese can cause blood glucose levels to be dangerously high, which can cause severe complications, including coma or death. Try to eat healthier and stick to a moderate exercise plan. It's never to late to change, and you can be successful no matter how many previous failed attempts you've had.

235.   It is important that you eat a lot of fiber in order to prevent diabetes. Fiber helps to prevent

diabetes by stabilizing your blood glucose levels. You can get fiber from certain foods such as whole grains, nuts, beans, seeds, fruits and vegetables. You can also take a fiber supplement.

236.   Do not rely on chocolate for a quick fix if your blood glucose levels drop. While most diabetics feel that this is a harmless remedy, it may actually have the opposite effect. The body absorbs fatty foods far more slowly, so you will notice a faster increase in glucose if you opt for a sweet, but fat-free, food.

237.   If you see ANY damage to the skin on your feet and you have Diabetes you must let your podiatrist know as soon as possible! He'll be able to tell you what to use to keep it clean and free of infection, and prescribe you an antibiotic cream or gel if necessary.

238.   There are many tasty snack ideas for diabetics; you just need to find the items you like. How about an apple with peanut butter? - weird but wondeful! A great alternative to peanut butter is almond butter, which is great on high-fiber crackers like ones made with rye flour. Or make your own snack mix out of a variety of nuts and dried fruit! Try grapes and feta cheese with balsamic vinegar.

239.   To decrease the effect sugars and carbohydrates have on your body, consume plenty of fiber. Fiber works as a sort of natural buffer that will help keep your blood sugar down even when you've eaten things that normally make it spike. If you've eaten something you shouldn't, a quick fiber rich snack can help counteract its effects.

240.   When you have diabetes, you probably have a team of doctors helping you out. You need to make sure that all of your doctors are on the same page, and are communicating with each other in a manner that puts your best interests first. Be assertive when it comes to your health care.

241.   Eating lots of fiber, offsets carbohydrates, as well as, sugars found in your system, which helps to maintain a healthy blood sugar level. Fiber can be found in many grains, vegetables, fruits and other foods. A healthy blood sugar level helps prevent diabetes and also, helps offset diabetic symptoms after you are already diagnosed. Make sure you have plenty of fiber in your diet.

242.   Drinking alcohol is something you need to be very careful with when you are diabetic. You

need to talk to your doctor to see if alcohol will affect your blood-glucose levels. If you are really not much of a drinker, it is best that you refrain from drinking at all.

243.   While it may be tempting to save yourself time and energy by eating out a lot of the time, you should only eat restaurant foods in moderation when trying to keep diabetes under control. Eating at home is much more cost effective and you have total control over what goes into each dish.

244.   A good tip for people dealing with diabetes is to never skip meals, especially breakfast. If you do not eat for several hours for whatever reason, your body relies on glucose released from your liver for energy. People with diabetes continue to produce glucose even when their body has had enough so make sure to eat something to let your liver know to stop producing glucose.

245.   Want a tasty treat that won't be forbidden by your doctor due to your Diabetes? Try nachos! Use a low fat cheese, low fat sour cream, homemade guacamole, and salsa, and you'll be getting a ton of nutrition with a burst of flavor. If you add some beans to the salsa you'll have an even healthier snack!

246.   If you're going to go a non-traditional route for your diabetes treatment, continue to be under the supervision of a doctor. Make sure to visit him at least every 3 months, so he can check your blood sugar levels, blood pressure and cholesterol. He should also test your organ functions, at the intervals he sets for you.

247.   It is possible to lower your blood sugar with exercise, so give it a try and see what it does for you. Make sure to test yourself immediately after you exercise to make sure your blood sugar has gone down to a level that is tolerable, otherwise you'll have to take your insulin.

248.   When traveling it is especially important to keep food with you. You may be strolling through a museum or shopping in an unknown area, and you could find that there is nothing healthy or appealing to eat. If you have your own snack it will at least tide you over until you can find something palatable.

249.   It can be hard to get enough exercise in when you're traveling, so plan for some hiking or walks to explore your new environment. Go swimming in the hotel pool, or even take an hour at the gym. Walking through the mall or a

museum can even serve as some extra movement.

250.   Make sure to visit the doctor if you have any of the risk factors involved with getting diabetes. Make an appointment as soon as possible if you are overweight, over the age of 45, have a very inactive lifestyle, or you have family with diabetes. The sooner you get the tested, the better chances you will have in catching the ailment early.

251.   A diet too high in protein can actually be harmful to diabetics. Some people think more protein is good, but studies have shown that too much animal protein can cause insulin-resistance, a factor in diabetes. Try to include proper amounts of protein, vegetables and carbohydrates to keep your diet healthy and well-balanced.

252.   To spot foods that may be an issue for you, keep track of what you eat in a log alongside of your glucose levels. After a while, you'll be able to notice the effect that certain foods have on you. This is a much better way to spot problematic foods than an elimination diet, and can also show you what foods benefit your health.

253.   It is important to control pre-diabetes with proper diet and exercise as well as keeping weight at normal levels. Studies show that even pre-diabetics are at risk of developing dangerous long-term damage from even mildly elevated blood sugar levels. These effects can be damaging even to the heart and circulatory system.

254.   If you're having trouble keeping yourself to a healthy Diabetic diet, don't change things up. Have a chicken night, a fish night, a lentil burger night, etc. so that you know what's supposed to happen on Thursday and can prepare for it. If you have something different every night you'll still have variation, but having a schedule will make you feel much less stress and you won't cave into temptation.

255.   To reduce the sugar in your diet, try using light or low-fat products when you cook. These products aren't just lower in fat- they also contain less sugar and sodium. This is a great way to continue to use things like peanut butter, sour cream, and cheese in your cooking.

256.   There are many signs and symptoms of diabetes, so it's possible to only have some of

them, or even none at all, and be diabetic. Some common symptoms encountered are tingling feet, high blood pressure, extreme lethargy, and an unquenchable thirst. Getting your blood-glucose levels checked once a year at your physical is absolutely imperative to a long, healthy life.

257.   Though this may seem like common knowledge for anyone who has ever taken medicine, many people for get to do it. As a Diabetic, you should always remember to take your medication! Only take medication prescribed by your doctor and only at interval that are safely prescribed for you.

258.   To make sure the carbohydrates you consume don't cause an issue for your body, eat them alongside protein. Protein will make sure your body absorbs the carbohydrates you eat slowly, which will help prevent dramatic changes to your blood sugar levels. Protein rarely increases blood glucose levels, and it's a great way to balance carbohydrates out.

259.   Making the switch to high fiber foods will help lower your risk for diabetes. Try to eat only whole grains, they are packed with fiber that allows your body to digest foods without getting

a spike in blood sugar which is what happens when you eat mostly refined carbs (white bread and any type of processed foods).

260.   Vinegar helps to keep blood sugar spikes at bay for diabetics who eat it during a meal. Some people actually recommend drinking it straight before you eat! I like to sprinkle it on a salad, or douse my vegetables in it. It's also great for marinating meats! It's extremely versatile.

261.   Going for a walk, jog, or run with your dog, is an excellent way to exercise and help keep your diabetes under control. It will also help your dog stay at a healthy weight, which can save you both heartache and money on vet bills. You'll motivate each other to keep going!

262.   You can get a free blood glucose meter from your pharmacy just by asking. They usually have coupons or rebates so that you can get the latest model at no cost, the caveat is that you'll be buying their brand of blood test strips for the rest of your life.

263.   Eating fresh, non-processed foods is an easy way for a diabetic to keep his or her weight in check and blood sugar stable. By shopping only the outside aisles of the grocery store you will

find you're not exposed to the processed sugary or carbohydrate-laden treats, that can lead to temptation.

264.   Diabetics should beware of caffeine as it can lead to potentially life-threatening blood pressure. Diabetes already has harmful effects on your organs, high blood pressure included, so you don't want to tax your body any more than it already is. Caffeine can lead in a massive spike in blood pressure after ingesting it, so just stay away from it completely.

265.   If you have Diabetes then it is important that you dry your feet carefully after a bath, shower, or a dip in the pool. Your feet will be more prone to getting infections, including fungal, so keeping them cool and dry can help prevent that from happening. Don't forget in between your toes!

266.   To better maintain your blood sugars, drink only water. Most other beverages are high in sugar, and diet soda can lead to dehydration, which can also cause your blood sugar levels to spike. Carrying around bottled water and drinking it regularly will help you keep your blood sugar levels where they're supposed to be.

267.	To make sure each meal you eat is balanced, divide your plate into sections. Devote half your plate to vegetables that are low in starch. Fill one quarter of the plate with healthy carbohydrates and the remaining quarter with a lean protein. This will make sure that your body gets everything it needs, keeping your diabetes in check.

268.	To save you and your doctor time, write down all of your questions about your diabetes. This way you will be prepared ahead of time and will not forget to ask anything that is important. You are dealing with your health, so don't be afraid to ask any question that you have.

269.	If you have diabetes, you should aim to drink as much water as you can. This particularly holds true when your blood glucose is elevated because high blood sugar can cause a large amount of urination. Therefore, you need to drink water to prevent yourself from dehydrating during this time.

270.	Do not eat foods that have a high level of salt if you have diabetes. These foods can raise your blood sugar levels along with raising your blood pressure, which can have negative consequences. There are many common foods that are made these days with little or not salt in them.

271.   Being diabetic does not mean that you must fully give up your favorite sweets, but it does mean that you must be more diligent in selecting and consuming them. To compensate for a sweet splurge, you may need to step up your exercise program, reducing your dietary intake of another sweet food, or taking more insulin.

272.   Diabetes related diseases are the second largest killer in The United States. This epidemic can be avoided with daily exercise and simple changes in diet. Cut out soda, candy and fatty meats and replace them with fruit, whole grains, and lean meats. This can add years to our life.

273.   Write up some quick emergency instructions for you to keep with you at all times. In these instructions makes sure to describe your care regimen in case you are rendered unconscious or unable to speak. This can be of great help to those who have a serious diabetic condition and can go into shock.

274.   As a diabetic, make sure you take your medications on time. Consult your physician for a time table to help calculate the appropriate

times for you to take your medication. Physicians may instruct you to take your pills before you eat or if you are also taking insulin, you may be required to take your pills at least thirty minutes before.

275.   If you are diabetic, watch for symptoms of hypoglycemia, or low blood sugar. These symptoms can include clammy hands, mouth numbness, and feeling extremely thirsty. Low blood sugar can lead to serious health complications if it is not immediately addressed. To counteract symptoms, eat a natural form of sugar and follow with a source of protein. Be sure to consult your doctors if symptoms do not improve.

276.   If you are trying to avoid diabetes, eat plenty of whole grains. Although no one has yet to pinpoint the exact reason why, whole grains have been show to lower your risk of developing diabetes. By including these grains in your diet, you will lower your risk of developing diabetes.

277.   The number one thing to keep in mind when you're diagnosed with Type II Diabetes is that it's not the end of the world! You will be able to live a long, healthy life with this condition as

long as you take the steps necessary to keep it under control.

278.   If you're having trouble getting the motivation to exercise after being diagnosed with Type II Diabetes, get in the game! Competitive sports are not only fun, but you have other people who rely on you to show up so that there are enough players for a game. Having them breathing down your neck will convince you to be on time!

279.   If your child is diagnosed with Diabetes, make keeping track of their blood sugar fun. Have a contest where they get a reward for doing their blood sugar on time every day for a certain number of days, like a trip to the toy store or an hour at the park.

280.   Hospitals will often have Diabetes clinics for local patients to attend, and they will have great advice for you. They'll give you tools to track your blood sugar, nutritional information for your diet plan, and even exercise tips. They can also be a great support group for you and will answer any questions that you might have.

281.   When you're on a plane it can be hard for a Diabetic to keep their feet moving. Try to do

little exercises while you sit, like moving your foot up and down or turning it in circles. Keep wiggling your toes to ensure your circulation gets blood right down to your tippy-toes.

282.   It is important that you have your cholesterol checked at least once a year if you have diabetes. Having diabetes increases your chances of developing high cholesterol, which can cause serious health problems like heart disease and stroke. There is a simple blood test called a fasting lipid profile that checks your cholesterol levels.

283.   If you are a diabetic make sure to carefully choose your lancing device. Pick one that maximizes comfort and minimizes pain especially since you will have to be testing very frequently. The better the device is, the less reluctant you will be with your blood sugar testings which will help improve the overall quality of your care.

284.   Smoking is unhealthy for anyone, but diabetics who do it are begging for trouble. Having this habit will expose you to a lot of unhealthy effects. Smoking actually increases your risk of getting type 2 diabetes as it makes you resistant to insulin.

285.   Clean out your pantry and fridge of all processed foods as well as foods high in sugar and trans fats. Eating trans fats and any food that has partially hydrogenated oils will increase your belly fat and put you at a higher risk for getting diabetes. These foods are not good for anyone to be eating, so it is best to toss them.

286.   When starting out on a journey, always bring along a bag that is insulated to carry diabetic supplies, such as insulin. You want to make sure that your insulin stays at the correct medium temperature. Using an insulated bad will protect you insulin from extreme hot or cold temperatures.

287.   With diabetes, it is important that you consult with professional help right away. This is important because there is plenty to be learned about the disease that only someone who specializes in it will know. Other than paid doctor visits, there are also toll free numbers that you can call for guidance.

288.   If you have diabetes and still crave sweets, just remember to eat them in moderation. It's a myth that diabetics can't eat any sugar at all --but it is true that diabetes means you need to

consume sugar with care. If you eat sweets, eat small amounts, and remember that the sweets count toward your carbohydrate tally for that meal.

289.   Another good way to prevent diabetes is to control your diet. Eating too many foods with a high glycemic index, which usually means foods with large amounts of simple sugars like candy or soda, can cause your cells to become less sensitive to insulin, which can cause diabetes. Eat less and save yourself the medical bills.

290.   A crucial tip for diabetics is to shed excess pounds. Dropping extra weight is a great way to help the body use insulin properly, reduce blood sugar levels and regulate blood pressure. A beneficial side effect is the increased energy levels typically experienced by those who achieve significant weight loss.

291.   If you need to sweeten your tea or coffee, but you have Diabetes, try using more natural sweeteners like honey or a sweetener and sugar substitute. These sweetener and sugar substitute can be found at many grocery stores today and is a plant extract, which is very sweet. It can even be found in a powdered form which mimics real sugar.

292.   If you want to eat healthier to help overcome your Diabetes, but you just can't stomach fish without some pops of flavor on it, try capers! They're like olives in their flavor, but smaller and zestier. You can sprinkle them on any type of fish, I like to also add some slices of Spanish onion, and they take the place of sauce.

293.   Diabetics should beware of caffeine as it can lead to potentially life-threatening blood pressure. Diabetes already has harmful effects on your organs, high blood pressure included, so you don't want to tax your body any more than it already is. Caffeine can lead in a massive spike in blood pressure after ingesting it, so just stay away from it completely.

294.   If you are the primary caregiver of a person with diabetes, you may need support also. You carry a heavy load caring for and making decisions for your loved one as well as monitoring their diet and lifestyle to keep them healthy. If you feel overwhelmed, ask for help. Your doctor can recommend respite care to give you a break, or even a nurse to help with care. You don't have to do it alone.

295.   Check to see if your grocery store puts out items that are close to their due date for clearance. Often, you can use things like ripe bananas for muffins or banana bread and you can find awesome sugar-free and low-carb recipes for both foods online. This can make for tasty and healthy treats, at a low cost, that any diabetic can enjoy!

296.   Diabetes is a complicated disease, which leads to many new precautions you'll need to take. One is to make sure that your dry ,cracked hands and feet remain moisturized. Your extremities will be at an increased risk of getting an infection, so ensuring dry skin doesn't crack open and let the germs in, is vital.

297.   Gestational diabetes can lead to Type II Diabetes later in life, so make sure the changes you implement during pregnancy continue after your baby is born. Having a healthy diet while breastfeeding is important, so keep eating cleanly throughout that time and afterward as well. Exercise will not only help you lose weight and tighten your skin back up, but it will also keep your blood sugar levels constantly normal.

298.   To keep from developing diabetes related circulation problems, regularly tap your feet!

Foot exercises will keep your blood moving even when you're stuck in a chair. Simply alternate lifting your heels or toes in the air while the other half of your foot remains on the floor. After time, this will become a habit, and keeping your circulation strong will be like second nature to you.

299.	Check your blood sugar often. This is very important if you are dealing with diabetes because you blood sugar can spike or get very low without you feeling any symptoms. You can buy a glucometer for less than $100.00 or you may be able to get it free from a diabetes educator.

300.	If you are diabetic, you need to be taking extra good care of your feet. More than half of all foot amputations are related to diabetes. Make sure you are cleaning them well, and not putting any extra strain on your feet. That means not standing for long periods of time, or doing anything to strenuous.

301.	If you have diabetes, you should avoid changing your medication without first talking to your doctor. It can be dangerous to experiment because your blood sugar can drop dangerously low by doing this. Therefore, you need to talk to your doctor, and find out what options he or she suggests for you.

302.   While some people view vacation as a chance to get away from all of their most pressing obligations, the same cannot be said of blood-glucose testing. Instead of entirely shirking your duties, you may be able to follow a more relaxed approach. You may be able to splurge on your eating habits, delay waking up for an early-morning glucose check, or testing as frequently.

303.   Due to the nature of diabetes and the circulation issues it can cause, you need to always pay attention to your feet and make sure that there are no infections developing. This is important because it is very easy to get an infection that could lead to the need for amputation if not caught in time or severe blood poisoning from dying skin tissue.

304.   When dealing with a child that has diabetes, make sure that the focus of conversations is not always about the disease. While it is important to keep them informed on any recent news about the disease or to obtain feed back from them about it, it is also important to engage in normal every day conversation to establish a sense of normalcy.

305.   People often throw the white flag up and confess that they are going to get diabetes in a couple years as the age. But the truth of the matter is many people can avoid diabetes completely even if it runs in their family. If a person lives a healthy life style and stays within the proper range for percent body fat they can live a life free of diabetes.

306.   If you want to eat healthier to help overcome your Diabetes, but you just can't stomach fish without some pops of flavor on it, try capers! They're like olives in their flavor, but smaller and zestier. You can sprinkle them on any type of fish, I like to also add some slices of Spanish onion, and they take the place of sauce.

307.   Educate your children in everything you learn about your Diabetes as they may face the same situation some day. It will be very helpful for them to see the journey you have taken and learn from it so that they can avoid mistakes when they grow up.

308.   Test your blood sugar before bed if you are Diabetic. It's important to eat something if your sugar is low to make sure you'll be okay over the long night until the morning. If your blood sugar

is just right then it's advisable to take a few bites of something to keep it up until you wake.

309.   Find out what your blood glucose target levels should be and ensure that you're meeting them. Diabetes control means knowing what you're up against, so keep a journal with your goal numbers listed so you can easily see how well you're doing every day. Once you have your blood glucose under control you'll feel immensely healthier!

310.   It is important for diabetics to take their insulin or other medications at the same time each day. Your doctor gave you this medication to control your diabetes and its symptoms and forgetting to take your medications or taking them at different times can raise your insulin or blood sugar.

311.   Research high glycemic index so that you can recognize them instantly. Breads, desserts, pastas, cereal, and even juices are products that are high in the glycemic index. Foods that have been overly processed can wreak havoc on blood sugar levels. Try eating fruits, veggies, meats, and fish instead.

312.   To spot foods that may be an issue for you, keep track of what you eat in a log alongside of your glucose levels. After a while, you'll be able to notice the effect that certain foods have on you. This is a much better way to spot problematic foods than an elimination diet, and can also show you what foods benefit your health.

313.   Even if you feel like your diabetes has gotten better, it is important not to stop taking your medications unless a doctor tells you it is alright to do so. The medications are most likely what is keeping your diabetes symptoms under control, so without them, your glucose or insulin levels could get out of control.

314.   There are many tasty snack ideas for diabetics; you just need to find the items you like. How about an apple with peanut butter? - weird but wondeful! A great alternative to peanut butter is almond butter, which is great on high-fiber crackers like ones made with rye flour. Or make your own snack mix out of a variety of nuts and dried fruit! Try grapes and feta cheese with balsamic vinegar.

315.   Lose weight. Bringing your weight down is not just a casual option; bringing down weight

will result in more stable blood sugar levels and less damage. Eat a healthy diet and exercise so that you can drop some weight and help your condition. Some obese diabetics who lose weight find they are no longer diabetic.

316.   To save you and your doctor time, write down all of your questions about your diabetes. This way you will be prepared ahead of time and will not forget to ask anything that is important. You are dealing with your health, so don't be afraid to ask any question that you have.

317.   There are more effective ways to measure where your blood sugar levels are at, than urine ketone testing. A high ketone level indicates that your blood contains 200 milligrams of sugar per deciliter. The ADA advises instead that diabetics rely on better and simpler methods of testing blood glucose levels, such as testing strips and finger sticks.

318.   If you are diabetic, you need to be taking extra good care of your feet. More than half of all foot amputations are related to diabetes. Make sure you are cleaning them well, and not putting any extra strain on your feet. That means not standing for long periods of time, or doing anything to strenuous.

319.   Be aware of what you are drinking. Many carbonated drinks and juices are made with high-fructose corn syrup, which is not good for anyone, let alone those with diabetes. These types of beverages are loaded with sugar (and thus, a lot of calories) that will leave you wanting more. Water should be your best friend!

320.   Watch out for trans-fats. Trans fats are found in any foods containing partially hydrogenated oils. These fats are dangerous for everybody, but diabetics are at extra risk. Trans fats cause increased amounts of fat around the waistline which has been linked to heart disease. They are also extremely high in calories and low in nutritional content.

321.   Watch your feet. More than half of all foot and leg amputations performed in the U.S. are related to diabetes. Diabetes can cause nerve damage and loss of feeling in your feet, known as Neuropathy. It is important for diabetics to check their feet often. You should watch for red spots and swelling, and keep your feet cared for by trimming your nails and wearing comfortable and supportive shoes.